The Vegan Muscle & Fitness Guide to Bodybuilding Competitions

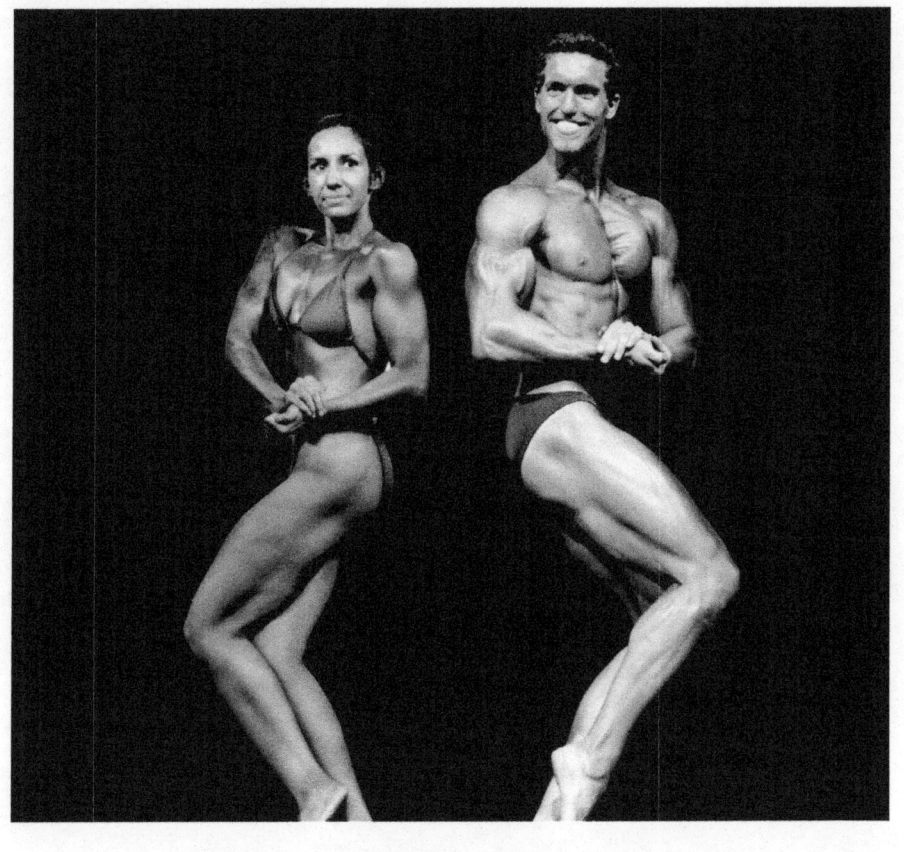

Left image by Brenda Carey, right image by Josh Avery

The Vegan Muscle and Fitness Guide to Bodybuilding Competitions

Derek Tresize, C.P.T.

Marcella Torres

First Printing: 2014

ISBN 978-1-312-42383-1

www.veganmuscleandfitness.com

Disclaimer

The fitness and nutrition information in this book is not intended to be a substitute for professional medical advice. Seek the advice of your physcician before implementing any of the nutrition or exercise suggestions contained within, and let common sense guide your actions!

Derek Tresize, Marcella Torres, publishers, printers, and others involved in this publication release themselves from any liability involving injury or loss as a result of applying the recommendations within this book.

Contents

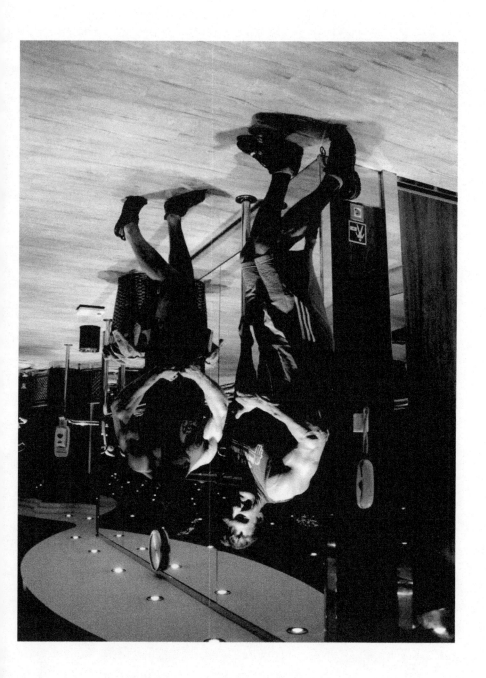

Foreword

By Robert Cheeke
Founder and President of Vegan Bodybuilding & Fitness, Champion Bodybuilder and Bestselling Author of *Vegan Bodybuilding & Fitness – The Complete Guide to Building Your Body on a Plant-Based Diet*

When I founded Vegan Bodybuilding & Fitness in 2002, the number of vegan bodybuilders I was aware of could have easily been counted on one hand, perhaps on just a few fingers. Resources to help an aspiring vegan athlete build muscle and burn fat and be competitive among omnivores in the sport of bodybuilding were essentially non-existent at the time. Therefore, everything I learned was through experimentation of trial and error. Some approaches worked well, others were not so effective. Regardless of the outcome of my efforts, I kept trying, kept learning and was striving for constant improvement to represent the vegan fitness lifestyle that was, and still is, so important to me.

Fast forward to 2014 and number of vegan athletes, and vegan bodybuilders, is impressive and growing rapidly by the day. We're still a minority in the sport of bodybuilding, but much like the sports of endurance running, mixed martial arts, and boxing, a vegan lifestyle could be commonplace in bodybuilding sooner than many might expect. While many tout the benefits of a plant-based diet to their increased aerobic capacity and quicker recovery after exercise, supporting their athletic pursuits, there are many more reasons to be on the right side of history by adopting a vegan lifestyle. Derek Tresize and Marcella Torres capture this very essence in The Vegan Muscle & Fitness Guide to Bodybuilding Contests. They provide a variety of meaningful reasons to adopt a vegan lifestyle in the first place and then clearly explain how a diet comprised of fruits, vegetables, grains, legumes, nuts and seeds provide optimal sources of macro and micronutrients, increased energy, enhanced recovery and greater control of your metabolic rate.

If this detailed and highly technical reference guide were available in the first decade of my competition days, I would likely have far more than two bodybuilding championships to my name, the number that Derek has already accumulated in far less time with stiffer competition. The reason why I am confident that sentiment is likely to be true is because of the step-by-step detailed nature of this guidebook to success. From precisely how to set your own personal physique goals based on your body type and work ethic, to tried and true formulas for building muscle and burning fat, to those somewhat complex and complicated steps that go into competing on stage as a competitive bodybuilder, Derek and Marcella have you covered. Had this reference been available years ago, we would have many more champion vegan bodybuilders in our growing community of successful vegan athletes today. It is inspiring to know that as a result of this publication, the future of bodybuilding will be changed for the better. If you have ever entertained the idea of becoming a physique competitor of any type, from bodybuilder to figure competitor, I am confident this resource will put you on the right path to success.

A plant-based diet and vegan lifestyle is more popular than ever before, and the opportunity to make a strong statement for veganism in athletes has never been greater than right now in the peak age of social media prevalence, which gives everyone a platform, everyone a voice, using tailor-made tools to get ideas worth spreading a lot of exposure.

Follow this guide to build your best physique and take it all the way to the stage if you feel compelled to join the ranks of those of us who have dared to be different, and to wear our vegan lifestyle on our sleeves as we represent an entire movement in our chosen sports. You will discover creative training and dieting strategies, will have a week by week guide to prepare you to be your best, and you will eat great food and have fun in your quest to represent veganism in athletics. You're in a far better position than I was when I got into this sport, simply because you have this book as guide and I didn't. We can't count the number of vegan bodybuilders on one hand anymore, and you might not even be able to count the number of vegan bodybuilders at your next competition on one hand either. That is what we call progress. Now is the time to use this resource to follow your passion and make it happen.

Wishing you all the very best in health and fitness.

Robert Cheeke, June 2014

About the Authors

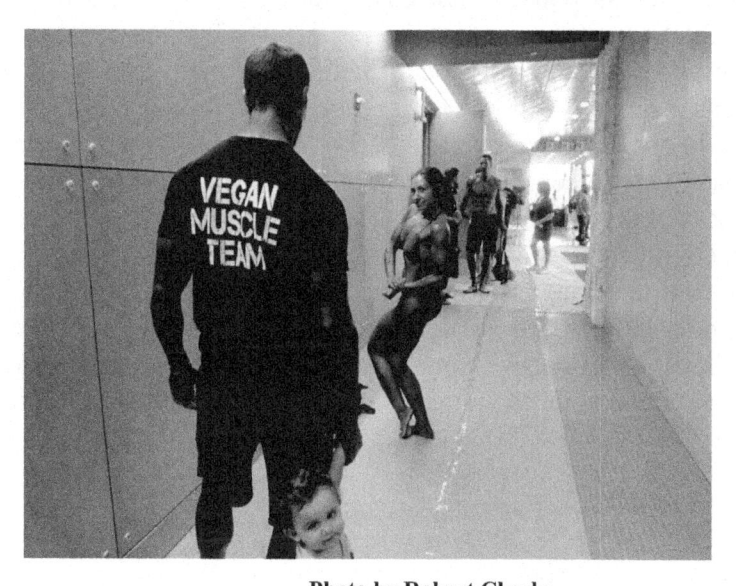

Photo by Robert Cheeke

Derek Tresize and Marcella Torres are the husband and wife team of competitive bodybuilders behind Vegan Muscle and Fitness at www.veganmuscleandfitness.com, where they have shared their training and nutrition tips, recipes and more since 2009. Owners of Richmond, Virginia's only plant-based personal training studio, Root Force Personal Training, the pair seeks to promote a fit and active plant-powered lifestyle and shatter the perception that strength and athleticism can't be achieved with a plant-based diet.

Derek is a three-time natural bodybuilding champion and pro bodybuilder with the World Natural Bodybuilding Federation. He is also an A.C.E. Certified Personal Trainer, is certified in Plant-Based Nutrition through the T. Colin Campbell Foundation and Cornell University, and holds a Bachelor of Science in Biology.

Marcella, formerly a professional mathematician, is now a competitive bodybuilder, professional meal planner, and professional dancer. She holds a Bachelor of Science in Applied Mathematics and Physics. Together they work with clients both internationally and locally helping everyone from new vegans to seasoned competitors build muscle and get lean with a whole-foods, plant-based diet. Their mission: to generate as many fit vegan role models as possible to get the message across that a plant-based diet isn't a handicap in the world of athletics – it's an advantage!

Derek and Marcella have been featured in many print and web publications such as *Vegan Health and Fitness* magazine, *Naked* magazine, *Vegan Lifestyle* magazine, *The Richmond Times-Dispatch*, *Style Weekly*, One Green Planet, The Daily Beet, Vegan Bodybuilding and Fitness, the *IDEA Fitness Journal*, Bodybuilding.com, BreakingMuscle.com, the television show *"What Would Julieanna Do?"*, and online radio programs such as *The Big Inside* on FTNS Radio. Both have been official sponsored athletes of Vegan Bodybuilding & Fitness and members of Team Plantbuilt, representing vegan athletes annually at the Naturally Fit Supershow in Austin, Texas.

Introduction

Do a Google search for the term "bodybuilding" combined with "gain", "lose", or "contest" and you will find that there are hundreds of books, articles, and trainers out there, ready to help you gain muscle or lose fat to prepare for a competition. The problem is that most of these resources will also tell you that to do so you need to eat animal products. We've written this comprehensive guide to vegan bodybuilding contest preparation to help you become living proof that nothing could be further from the truth! A plant-based diet will give you the advantage, allowing you to recover faster, giving you higher energy levels, and, most importantly, keeping you healthy and vital inside and out.

Being a visibly fit and healthy vegan is also a surprisingly powerful form of activism. A fit appearance can be a marketing tool: the slick advertising that draws people in and primes them to hear you out as you make the case for a vegan lifestyle! It was this realization that prompted us to devote ourselves full-time to the health and fitness field, hoping to help more role models take up the cause.

After fielding hundreds of questions through our blog Vegan Muscle and Fitness, at vegetarian festivals and speaking events, and from personal training clients at our Richmond, Virginia studio, we've realized that it's time for a definitive guide to preparing for competitions as a vegan athlete! Years of training and competition experience have been condensed into this book, offering the nitty-gritty on everything from calculating lean body mass to choosing a competition suit. This includes seven years of experience training hundreds of clients, both competitive athletes and those who simply want to improve their physique, online and in person, from all over the world. It includes our own experiences as bodybuilding competitors, over our tenure as members of the PlantBuilt vegan bodybuilding team, and as sponsored athletes for Vegan Bodybuilding and Fitness. Add to this massive amount of empirical data our backgrounds in science and research and the result is a technical manual with all of the mysteries of muscle gain and fat loss decoded into instructions that you can immediately put into practice, grounded in the latest research.

Are you ready to be a role model? Great, then let's get started!

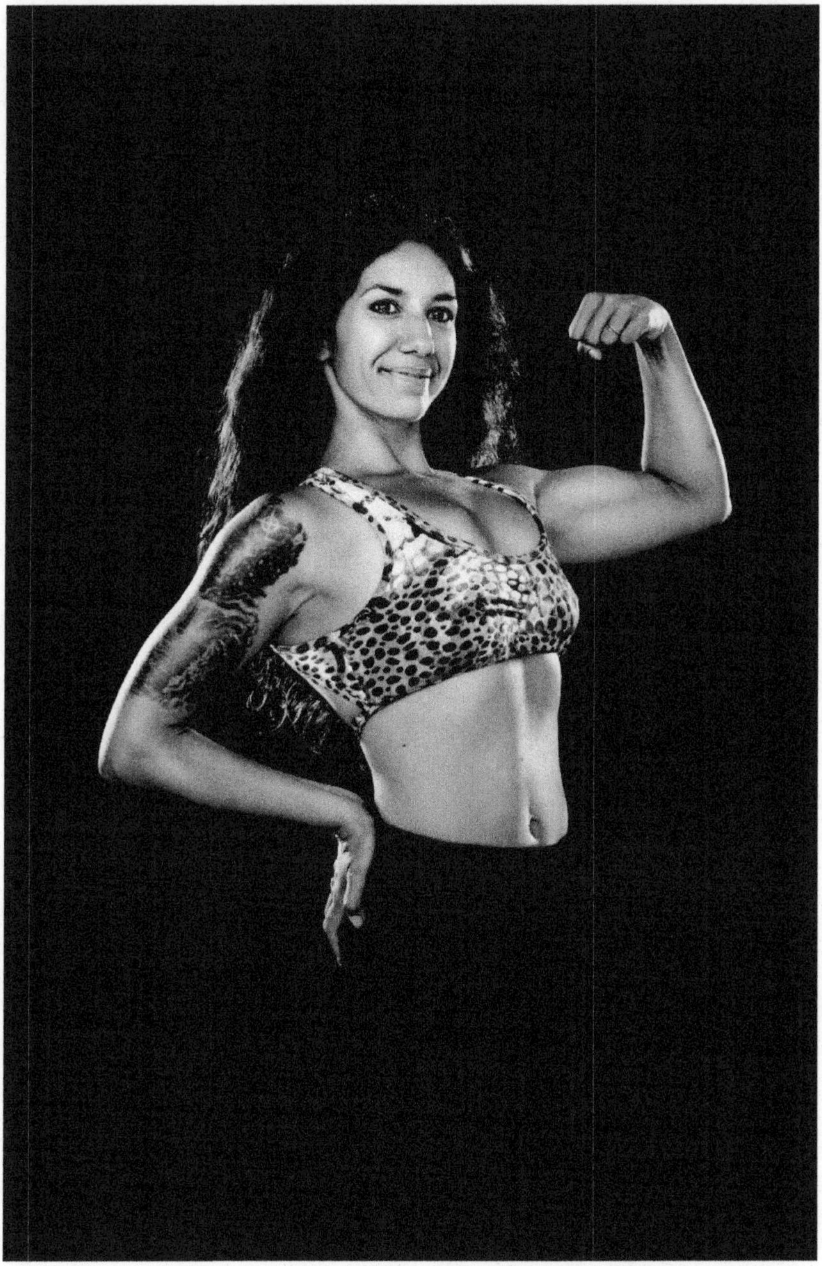

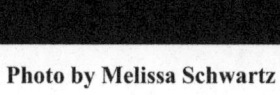

Photo by Melissa Schwartz

Section 1: The Off-Season

The off-season describes that time of year, usually November through March, when there are no contests to prepare for and athletes are focusing on building muscle rather than burning body fat. This phase is also commonly referred to as the "bulking" phase.

This is a favorite time of year for most physique athletes because they are spending less time at the gym, focusing on strength and muscle gain rather than fat loss, and they have eased their dietary restrictions. Since it begins with relaxation and recovery after the contest season, many competitors go in without a plan and end up falling behind on their physique goals or, worse, gaining far too much fat. It is important to remember that the off-season is a vital part of your competitive year and that in addition to gaining muscle and strength, you must prioritize maintaining low body fat and a robust metabolism. It is far better to put the time in up front, during your off-season, than to play catch-up during the more stressful phases of contest preparation!

Chapter 1: Setting Goals

The very first step to competitive bodybuilding is putting pen to paper and setting some specific, measurable goals. Start with your body as it is right now. Do a weigh-in in the morning on an empty stomach, measure your current body fat level using calipers (search "how to use body fat calipers" for video tutorials), take photos of your body in minimal clothing from all four sides, and even take circumference measurements. Write it all down and record the date. This is your starting point. Now it's time to figure out your targets.

Using your current weight and body fat, calculate your lean body mass this way:

Body Fat Mass = Body Weight x (% Body Fat)/100
Lean Body Mass = Body Weight - Body Fat Mass

For example, if you had a current body weight of 180 lbs and a body fat percentage of 15%, you would calculate

Body Fat Mass = 180 lbs x (15%)/100 = 27 lbs

and

Lean Body Mass = 180 lbs - 27 lbs = 153 lbs

This is what your body would weigh with absolutely no body fat (an impossibility, of course, but a useful reference point). Before you start looking at possible show dates, your goal is to build as much lean body mass as you can while simultaneously targeting a healthy body fat percentage. If you are currently overweight or obese this will involve training to gain muscle mass while adjusting your nutrition and cardiovascular exercise protocol to reduce body fat to a more reasonable level. If, on the other hand, you are already very lean this will involve taking time to diligently increase your calories while training to gain as much muscle as possible and limiting gains in body fat to no higher than your targeted percentage. While the starting points of each individual athlete will vary, no one should begin dieting down for a show until they are at a healthy level of body fat with ample lean body mass. The sport of bodybuilding is all about maximizing lean body mass while minimizing body fat and so, to a lesser extent, are all of the other categories (physique, figure, bikini, etc.).

Body Types

When planning your goals and their subsequent time frames, it is important to keep your somatotype, or body type, in mind. There are three general somatotypes, and while most individuals are a blend of two or more rather than being easily categorized by just one, the definitions are helpful for building expectations about how your body will respond to diet and exercise, and how quickly.

Ectomorphs are thin individuals characterized by narrow hips and shoulders, long limbs with small joints, and a very fast metabolism. An ectomorph has very low body fat levels and not too much muscle mass. These individuals are often described as lanky, wiry, tall, or lean. They can generally eat a lot of calorie dense foods without gaining much if any body fat, but they have a very hard time accumulating muscle mass, and they require a lot of extra calories to increase their body weight even a little.

Since an ectomorph's main struggle will be to accumulate muscle mass in the off-season and keep it during a contest diet, this should be the main focus of his or her diet and training. Lifting should be centered on heavy compound exercises at a moderate to low volume (not too many sets and reps per workout) in order to stimulate muscle gain without burning too many calories. Likewise, cardio training should be kept to a minimum in order to conserve muscle mass and not burn too many calories. An ectomorph will usually only have to do the very lowest amount of cardio before a contest, while also consuming nearly their maintenance calories (calories required to maintain current weight) to prevent muscle loss. Some schools of thought believe an ectomorph should eat a higher carbohydrate, lower fat diet than the other somatotypes, and also that due to their narrow frame and small joints they are more likely to suffer injuries, but this may be mere conjecture.

Mesomorphs are naturally strong, athletic looking individuals characterized by broad shoulders, medium sized joints and hips and a moderately fast metabolism. A mesomorph will generally have low to normal body fat levels, and is able to gain muscle and lose fat fairly easily. Mesomorphs are often 'natural athletes' who can usually lift more weight, sprint faster and jump higher than their peers.

A mesomorph will not have to be as careful about his or her training as either an ectomorph or an endomorph due to the fact that his or her body will respond well to almost any stimulus, but should still be mindful not to eat too much unhealthy, calorie dense food to prevent excess bodyfat gain.

Endomorphs are naturally thick, heavyset individuals characterized by wide hips, medium to broad shoulders, thick joints and a stockier frame than the other somatotypes. Endomorphs are the most likely individuals to be overweight and have a hard time losing body fat due to their slow metabolisms. However, an endomorph can also usually gain muscle mass and strength fairly quickly, he or she will just have a hard time losing bodyfat when they prepare for a contest. An endomorph will likely need to eat a more closely monitored diet and maintain a moderately high level of cardio all year round to prevent excess body fat gain, and in their training it is also often recommended to train with higher volume (more sets and reps) in order to increase caloric expenditure there as well.

Some schools of thought believe that endomorphs should eat a higher fat, lower carbohydrate diet due to their slower metabolisms, and that they are more resistant to injury because of their thicker, sturdier joints but, as with ectomorphs, this is likely conjecture.

Very few individuals fall squarely into just one of the somatotypes, as we are all unique and are often a blend of two if not all three to some extent. For example, Derek is an ecto-mesomorph – he has a fast metabolism and and requires a lot of food just to maintain his weight, but is naturally pretty strong and gains muscle much more easily than a purely ectomorphic individual would. Also, your body can and will change over time. With consistent, healthy eating and hard training everyone's body will become more like that of a bodybuilder's, and with less effort. The first time Derek set a goal of breaking 190 pounds of body weight he had to eat 7000 calories per day to reach it, whereas now he can easily meet or surpass this weight with around 4000 calories per day. With the hard training and consistent eating his body has become less ectomorphic and more mesomorphic.

There are an infinite variety of bodies out there, so be careful when reading these descriptions not to lump yourself into one over the others and base your entire diet and training philosophy on that. The best way to learn about your body will always be through trial and error, so take time, take notes and see what works for you.

Gaining Muscle

The details of developing your own mass-gaining plan will be outlined in the off-season section of this book, but for the sake of setting goals we will cover some basic parameters here. The rate at which you can gain muscle will depend on your genetics, your somatotype, and how long you have already been training. A beginner with average genetics will often make fantastic progress in the first year of training, but an advanced athlete who already has substantial muscle mass and training experience will have to fight for every additional ounce. Keeping that in mind, a very rough estimate of the rate at which someone can gain maximal muscle with minimal body fat is about 2 to 5 pounds per month. Some of this weight will always be body fat. Even if your body fat started out at 18% and remained so after gaining 5 pounds, 18% of that 5 pounds would have come from gained body fat. This is still an excellent rate of muscle gain. As with anything in the body, this process is not linear so you can expect to witness rapid gains as well as plateaus, but the above rate can serve as a rule-of-thumb over the long run. You can now look at your starting point and determine a time frame for gaining a specific amount of weight and muscle mass.

For example, let's say your mass gain goal is to add eight pounds of lean body mass before you pick your contest and begin dieting. Eight pounds may not sound like a lot, but it can make a substantial difference! If you have some weightlifting experience, average genetics, and are willing to put 100% effort into your diet and training you can reasonably expect to gain about ½ pound of lean mass per week. This gives you 16 weeks, or 4 months, to reach your goal of 8 pounds.

You now have a reasonable time frame to work with. If you find your progress is a little faster or slower than anticipated you can always adjust your time frame after a few weeks of evaluation. Just remember: slower is always better!

Losing Fat

Similarly, if you have a body fat loss goal you can calculate a time frame in which to meet it. Even for the quintessential endomorph shedding body fat is actually easier, although more unpleasant, than gaining muscle. So don't be daunted by the amount of fat you need to lose. Just as there is an expected average range of muscle gain over time there is a range of fat you can expect to lose over time. You may have heard of the benchmark of about 2 pounds of fat loss per week as being optimal, and that's about right. Someone who begins this process with a very high level of body fat will likely witness faster progress, especially at first, than someone who is already fairly lean. You may also have heard that the last few pounds are the hardest; unfortunately, it's true!

Another important aspect of fat loss to consider is body composition. If you're just getting into training you will be gaining muscle mass almost as fast as you lose body fat. This is why some athletes become discouraged that their weight isn't budging even though they may be gaining strength and simultaneously losing inches. The best way to maintain an objective view of your progress is to regularly check your body composition along with your weight. By monitoring not just changes in pounds on the scale but lean body mass you will be able to see if you are in fact shedding body fat even when your weight remains unchanged.

Let's say Bob begins training at 25% body fat and 204 pounds with the target of beginning a contest diet when he reaches 15% body fat. By calculating Bob's current lean body mass at 204 pounds (204 x 25%/100) we see that he has a lean body mass of 153 pounds. Now, in order to maintain the same lean body mass at 15% body fat, Bob would set his target weight at 180 pounds and aim to lose about 24 pounds of fat (see example calculation on page 1). With an average weight loss of 1.5 pounds per week, Bob can expect to reach his goal in about 16 weeks.

After 16 weeks, Bob has only dropped to 187 pounds and, frustrated, measures his body composition. It's 15%, just as he'd planned! What happened? Bob forgot to take into account that 16 weeks is plenty of time for an untrained person to gain several additional pounds of muscle and he gained 6 pounds of lean body mass in addition to reaching his fat loss goal! This example illustrates the importance of tracking your body fat percentage and lean body mass rather than weight alone.

Bodybuilding Divisions

Listed below are the different divisions with a description of the desired physique for each, and the expected body fat ranges for athletes.

Bodybuilding: Muscular. Male body fat should be around 3-4%, female around 6-10%.

Physique: Lean and athletic with a balanced build. Male body fat should be around 5-7%, female around 8-12%.

Figure: Lean and fit, with bigger shoulders and leaner legs. Female body fat should be around 8-12%.

Bikini: Curvy, sexy, and lean without being 'shredded'. Female body fat should be around 10-15%.

These body fat ranges will tell you how long you will need to diet, but deciding how much time to dedicate to muscle gain is a bit harder to estimate. My suggestion is to visit a local bodybuilding competition and observe the category you plan to compete in; specifically, the height or weight class you will likely be in when in contest condition. Look at how the judges place the competitors and compare yourself to the winners of your class. If you feel that you have a comparable amount of muscle mass you might dedicate as little as 3 to 6 months to gaining lean mass but if, on the other hand, you have a long way to go to get mass comparable to what you see on stage don't be afraid to plan ahead by as much as 12 to 18 months before you step on stage.

Allow yourself enough time to avoid feeling rushed and anxious so that you can enjoy witnessing the changes in how you look and feel. You can always re-assess your progress and choose an earlier or later show date. So have fun!

Setting a Body Fat Ceiling

There are two basic components of successful muscle gain: a calorie surplus and an appropriate training stimulus. There are many different philosophies about off-season nutrition, and the most common one goes something like this: "You gotta eat big to get big, so anything goes! Eat as much as you can of whatever you want and lift big!"

That will certainly cause you to gain weight, but how much of it will be muscle and how much will be fat? We suggest a more conservative approach: eat a fairly small caloric surplus composed of almost all clean food, train hard and effectively, and, unless you're an extreme ectomorph, maintain some cardiovascular exercise even in the off-season. You will gain weight at a slower rate but a very high percentage of the weight will be lean muscle, saving you the grueling work of sloughing off the excess fat later. You may even lose some body fat, keeping you looking great in the off-season and within striking distance of contest condition year round.

An important tool to minimize fat gain is a body fat ceiling. This is an upper limit of body fat to stay below during your muscle gain phase. What that number is will depend on the amount of fat you begin with, how aggressively you want to gain muscle mass, and how much time remains until the beginning of your diet if you've already selected a contest. As a general rule, we advise clients to keep their body fat in the normal and healthy range during the off-season and avoid getting into the overweight range, which is above 15% for men and above 25% for women. If you are already well below these numbers, a lower ceiling makes sense, and if you are above them then we recommend trying to get into the healthy range even during the off-season.

Staying lean and maintaining some cardio in the off-season may not be as fun as pigging out and lifting big, but it offers some serious advantages. Off-seasons are more lax in general, so you can certainly still enjoy meals out on occasion and even some sweet treats, but keeping your body fat ceiling in mind will ensure that things don't get out of control and will make you a much more effective competitor!

Staying Fit in the Off-Season Q&A

Q: But I thought the off-season was the fun part! Why do I need to stay so lean?

You don't, actually. Plenty of competitors pile on the body fat when they aren't competing and still manage to get into show condition consistently, but here are some benefits to staying lean:

A shorter, easier diet. The longer and more restricted your pre-contest diet needs to be, the more muscle you are likely to lose and the more worn out you will be on stage. Why make the process any harder than it already is?

Improved performance and health. Gaining too much fat is never a good thing for an athlete, with the possible exception of a sumo wrestler. If you are overweight it will be harder to get through your intense workouts, it will take you longer to recover, and your stamina for cardiovascular exercise will suffer. Being overweight is also negatively affects your long-term health.

Gaining too much fat may actually hinder muscle gain. Yes, more food in generally means more muscle on your frame but in addition to making it harder to train intensely, excess fat causes a number of physiological changes that can hinder gains. It drops testosterone levels and increases estrogen production, leading to less muscle gain, a slower metabolism, and more fat storage.

Excess fat increases insulin resistance. Maintaining insulin sensitivity allows your body to quickly and effectively shuttle nutrients to hungry muscle cells with every insulin release. As your resistance goes up with your body fat, more and more insulin must be released in order to absorb nutrients from your food, keeping your muscles from getting fed efficiently. Also, the more insulin you release, the easier it is to gain more fat.

You will look and feel better year-round and continue to be a positive role model. We don't know about you, but we prefer looking fit. **It motivates us to train harder when we feel like we look good, we're able to jump into other physical activities with ease, and we don't miss out on unexpected opportunities like photo shoots that would be out of the question if we were completely out of shape.** Even more importantly, we consider ourselves representatives of plant-based nutrition at all times. Our vegan message shirts get us a little more scrutiny at the gym, and when we look fit and lift strong - that's a good thing!

Q: Do I really need cardio in the off-season? I hate it!

Yes, most bodybuilders hate long bouts of cardiovascular exercise and look forward to the off-season as a break from the tedium, but eliminating it entirely is a mistake. Here's why:

Maintaining some regular cardio will help you train harder. Just as staying lean helps you train harder, staying in good cardio shape does, too, and will therefore help you build more muscle. Don't believe me? Try doing a heavy set of squats, lunges, or deadlifts for more than 10 repetitions - how even is your breathing afterwards? Now repeat for four more sets with one minute of rest in between sets. See what I mean?

Cardio can improve recovery. Spending 20 to 30 minutes a couple of times per week moving your whole body and increasing your breath and heart rates will get a larger volume of blood moving past your sore muscles, delivering oxygen and nutrients and removing unwanted waste products. Better recovery = better workouts = more muscle.

Cardio makes it easy to stay lean. And we just discussed all the benefits of that!

Eating Clean

Just as having a body fat ceiling is important, striving to eat clean, healthy whole plant foods the majority of the time yields many rewards. In fact, staying lean and eating clean are two sides of the same coin; good luck achieving the former without the latter! As a vegan you are probably already aware of how food can affect how you think, feel, and perform and it's no surprise that these effects are especially important to understand for the competitive athlete. Here are some great reasons to eat clean year round:

- Eating healthy whole foods will provide your body with all of the nutrients it needs to fuel performance and the antioxidants it needs to recover faster.
- It's a lot easier to stay lean eating large amounts of healthy food than otherwise. Who gets fat from too many beans? And again, when it's time to diet, why make it any harder? In fact, the transition from "bulking" to "cutting" will hardly be noticeable if all you are doing is gradually reducing the amounts of the foods that already make up your daily menu.
- Healthy food is better for your long-term health (this is a no-brainer!). The off-season could be considered to be any time you're not actively preparing for a contest, and that's probably most of the time, so be mindful that how you are eating now is really how you eat *most of the time* rather than a temporary vacation from thoughtful, nutritious eating.
- As an athlete, especially a vegan athlete, you're a role model! Do you want your friends, family, and gym buddies to think that vegans need to eat junk food and meat and dairy analogues in order to be satisfied? Or would you rather demonstrate that you could get optimal nutrition simply by eating whole plant foods?

Jacked on Junk Food?

An alternative approach to eating healthy year-round is the "if it fits your macros" (IIFYM) method. This is an anything goes style of eating that allows any foods in your meal plan as long as, overall, you are hitting your target calories and grams of protein, carbohydrates, and fat every day. There are some very successful competitors out there, even pros, who use this method successfully demonstrating that it's possible to build muscle and get into show condition eating a lot of junk food. Our question is: is it optimal? Given the reasons we've listed above for eating clean, we're confident that, in the long run, the answer is 'no'.

Chapter 2: Training Strategies

The primary objectives of the off-season for a physique athlete are gaining lean muscle mass and increasing your metabolic rate. To meet these goals, some specific training methods can be employed to maximize your results. Let's go over some important background information that will make it clear why some training methods are superior to others.

First, what makes muscles grow? Skeletal muscle is an extremely complex and specialized tissue and the answer to this question is likewise very complicated. To put it simply, addressing these five variables stimulates muscle growth:

1. **Mechanical stress:** the amount of weight you train with, often referred to as 'intensity'.
2. **Metabolic stress:** the total number of exercises, sets, and reps, which is often referred to as 'volume'.
3. **Proper nutrition:** a caloric surplus, adequate macronutrients, and leucine levels.
4. **Adequate rest and recovery time.**
5. **Progressive overload:** an increased workload over time.

A well-designed training program will incorporate at least three of the five variables listed above, finding the perfect balance of each for a particular athlete. In addition, there are some training techniques of interest to all athletes because they employ several of the above variables at once, and without fail the champions have mastered them. Including compound exercises in your routine is one of them.

Compound Exercises

A compound exercise is any exercise that uses multiple muscle groups and moves multiple joints. Some quintessential compound exercises are squats and deadlifts and it's no coincidence that they are each sometimes called the 'king of lifts' in terms of gaining muscle size and strength. Other commonly used exercises are bench press, overhead press, barbell rows, pull-ups, dips, lunges...the list goes on! Why do these exercises seem to work so well for everyone?

- They provide ample amounts of both the mechanical and metabolic stress required for muscle growth
- They allow you to lift more weight because you are recruiting multiple muscle groups at once
- A tremendous metabolic response is elicited when all of those muscle groups are worked simultaneously, using large amounts of calories and oxygen, generating a lot of waste products like lactic acid, and thereby causing a big hormone response

Compound exercises hit numbers one and two on the list of muscle-growth strategies hard; this is why they're an essential part of your training routine, and why they're so hard! Just remember, if it doesn't challenge you, it doesn't change you!

Sets and Repetitions

Just as there are exercises that will yield the greatest results in the least amount of time during your off-season, there is also an ideal range for the sets and reps that should be performed for muscle gain by most athletes, most of the time. Once again, these ranges relate directly to numbers one and two on our list: mechanical stress and metabolic stress. To induce mechanical stress you generally want to stay within the 3 to 6 rep range, and for metabolic stress you should perform at least 15 reps. Assuming that you are always lifting as much weight as you can at the above rep ranges, either range option will provide excellent stimulus for muscle growth.

However, there is a rep range in which you can elicit some of each type of stress and increase your training efficiency. It's the rep range that the most successful physique athletes use the most often: 8

to 12 reps. A maximal effort set of 10 reps, exactly midrange, allows you to train with enough weight for good mechanical stress at a high enough rep range to generate some serious metabolic stress, especially with compound exercises. How many reps you will use on most of your sets will vary based on your goals and somatotype, but sets of eight to twelve maximal effort reps with compound exercises will elicit the biggest gains in strength and muscle mass in the shortest period of time.

How many sets to do per muscle group in a single workout can vary substantially depending on the muscle group in question, your training frequency, and who you talk to. As a general rule, you should strive to train each muscle with between 10 and 24 total sets per workout, with the higher number of sets being allotted to larger muscle groups, and to any muscle groups you are training less frequently. For example, if you are training a large muscle group such as your back once per week, it is completely reasonable to perform 24 total sets - with 4 sets each of 6 different exercises. However, if you are training a large muscle group at a higher frequency, such as 3 times per week, or training a small muscle group like biceps, then 10 total sets per training session would be more than sufficient for each muscle group, and more would likely be overkill.

Now, does this mean you should train exclusively with compound exercises in the eight to twelve rep range only? Not necessarily. Isolation exercises that work one muscle and one joint have their place in a well-rounded program, as do a variety of rep ranges. Many lifters have naturally dominant muscle groups that will overpower some compound exercises, leaving other targeted muscle groups under-stimulated. For example, Derek has a strong mind-muscle connection with his back and is able to use it very effectively on back exercises. The downside of this is that, unlike most trainees, his arms get very little stimulation from training his back and if he wasn't careful to include plenty of isolated arm exercises he would have a very disproportionate physique - a thick torso with little stick arms! The issue of dominant muscle-groups is common among bodybuilders: some have dominant triceps that prevent them from getting chest stimulation from bench presses, others overuse their biceps when training their backs, and so on. The solution to this problem lies in isolation exercises.

It will take a lot of time training and careful observation of its effects before you learn which of your muscle groups are dominant and which are stubborn and take additional effort to provoke growth. In the meantime, it's a good idea for a less experienced athlete to include one to two isolation exercises per muscle group, per workout, just to ensure that every part of your body is getting adequate attention.

Training Frequency

Another consideration when designing your training routine is its frequency. How often you work each muscle can have a huge impact on your progress. The most popular training frequency right now is once per week for each muscle group, but this wasn't always the case.

In the 'Golden Era' of bodybuilding, when Arnold Schwarzenegger was competing, it was common for bodybuilders to train each muscle group 2 to 3 times every week and this higher frequency training has played a major role in producing champions.

What do Arnold, Lee Haney, and Ronnie Coleman all have in common? They've each won the most prestigious bodybuilding title, Mr. Olympia, seven or eight times (far more than any other competitors), *and* they all trained each muscle group 2 to 3 times every week. Other famous past bodybuilders to utilize high frequency have been Frank Zane, Franco Columbu, Lou Ferrigno, and Sergio Olivia. This is virtually every top bodybuilder from the golden age, when many believe bodybuilders looked their best. A modern bodybuilder who utilizes twice per week frequency is none other than three-time Mr. Olympia Phil Heath. In addition, many top natural bodybuilders train with higher than once-per-week frequency for certain muscle groups or their whole body such as Marin Daniels, Doug Miller, and Dr. Layne Norton. Even the Godfather of Vegan Bodybuilding, Robert Cheeke, cites multiple daily sets of pushups and crunches as one of the secrets to his bodybuilding success. And Derek has seen by far the greatest gains when he trains each muscle group two to three times per week.

Now, why does high frequency training produce such excellent results? It's the same principle as that employed by any other type of athlete, from dancers to martial artists: if you want your body to adapt to something, provide it the signal to do so as often as possible. In other words, practice!

A study published in the August 2000 edition of the *Journal of Strength and Conditioning Research* titled 'Comparison of 1 Day and 3 Days Per Week of Equal-Volume Resistance Training in Experienced Subjects' demonstrated one possible reason when it compared two groups performing the same exact training program either in one workout per week, or divided into three workouts per week. By the end of the study the three-times-per-week group had gained significantly more muscle mass and strength than the once per week group, performing the exact same workout! They performed the exact same amount of work, but they gave their bodies the message to grow three times a week rather than once.

Another factor at play is illustrated by a quote from the Exercise Science Department of Florida Atlantic University: "Strength and growth are related to total training volume, not exercise-induced muscle damage". By training more often, your volume over time will be much greater. Training a muscle group once per week with high volume may amount to 25 total sets for that muscle each week, but training that same muscle with the moderate volume of 15 sets twice per week will result in 30 total sets per week, and we guarantee you will be able to train with more focus and intensity for 15 sets in one workout than you will for 25. If the same amount of work spread out with more frequency can yield superior results, imagine what greater total volume and a higher relative intensity can do, especially when you consider the cumulative effect over a year's time!

In fact, we consistently see the fastest progress in our clients seeking to gain muscle mass when we implement a total body routine that trains each muscle group every workout. In this workout plan, we select the top three to four exercises for each muscle group (for example: squats, lunges and leg press for legs) then write three to four separate workouts with one exercise for each muscle group therein. That way there is still a variety of exercises to provide a diverse stimulus, but each exercise can be trained at maximal intensity since it is always done when that muscle group is fresh - providing three to four intense training stimuli per muscle group every week. This is an excellent plan for a novice to follow for rapid gains in size and strength, but as a lifter gets more advanced, a split routine will become necessary to allow for a greater volume of training per session, as well as slightly longer recovery intervals.

There are limits to how frequently you should train, of course. You can't train every muscle group with brutal intensity every single day or you'd never be able to recover and adapt, and you would likely become injured. And that is the one drawback we've found with high frequency training: you are more likely to get injured unless you keep your intensity in check and ensure optimal recovery. Nothing will derail your progress like an injury, so how much frequency is too much? That is very much an individual question, but as a general rule we don't recommend training a given muscle group more than three times per week. In addition to this, the more often you train a muscle, the more you should err on the side of training short of muscle failure and doing less volume at each session, or at least alternate between brutal sessions and easier ones. Bodybuilding is a sport of *recovering* from weight training, not just weight training, so you need to ensure you are recovering as much as possible between sessions. To do this, don't train to failure on every set or even every workout, and if you've been training intensely and consistently for 4 to 6 weeks, don't be afraid to take a deloading week and train with 30 to 50% less weight than you normally do for each exercise. When using higher frequency, it's important to keep an eye on your recovery to avoid over training. If your energy is consistently low, your strength and performance are decreasing instead of increasing, and/or you are suffering from chronic muscle soreness you are likely overtraining and need to reduce all training substantially for several weeks to allow full recovery. Unless a muscle has been inadvertently over trained, it typically only needs 48 to 72 hours to recover between workouts, so valuable training opportunities may be lost by training with less frequency. However, the deciding factor will always be what works best for you and for your body.

High Frequency Programs

There are many ways to structure a high frequency program, but following are some tried and true examples. Keep in mind that there are thousands of possible routines that can be created from the basic structures listed below! A great way to find more detailed examples, if you find yourself overwhelmed with exercises to choose from, is to simply search the Internet for templates; for example, searching "push/pull/legs" will give you many templates from which to craft your own routine that fits your own preferences and limitations.

Three Day Splits

Push/Pull/Legs
Chest and Back/Shoulders and Arms/Legs
Back and Hamstrings/Chest and Arms/Shoulders and Legs

Two Day Splits

Upper/Lower
Total Body Push/Total Body Pull

Total Body, Two to Four Times Weekly

Here is one example of how such a routine could be structured:

Day 1
    Bench Press
    Barbell Row
    Overhead Press
    Squat
    Barbell Curl
    Hanging Leg Raise

Day 2
    Incline Bench Press
    Pull-ups
    Power Clean
    Leg Press
    Dips
    Crunches

Day 3
    Deadlift
    DB Pullover

Seated Arnold Press

DB Lunges

Close Grip Bench Press

Hanging Leg Raise

Day 4

DB Bench Press

DB Row

Barbell Shrug

Romanian Deadlift

Preacher Curl

Crunches

Off-Season Cardio

Unless you're an extreme ectomorph, doing some cardio in the off-season is actually advantageous. It keeps your fat gains to a minimum and improves your performance in the gym, which in turn leads to better workouts and then to better gains. There are many types of cardio out there to choose from, but which types are optimal when you are trying to gain muscle?

A lot of research has gone into answering that question and the findings are conclusive. The shorter, the more intense, and the more physically similar to compound exercises your cardio activity is, the more it will stimulate your body to burn fat, produce anabolic hormones, and improve cardiovascular performance. All of these spell better results for your off-season. Such exercises include:

- Sprinting, which is similar to jumping, lunging, and squatting
- Cycling, which is similar to squatting
- Rowing, which is similar to weightlifting rows and deadlifts

Exercises such as these will stimulate many large muscle groups through a long range of motion, so performing them at a high level of intensity actually causes a physiological response similar to strength training and can actually cause some muscle gains in their own right! In order to keep the intensity appropriately high, it's important to keep the work intervals short and to provide enough recovery between them to ensure that the following intervals remain as intense as possible. This style of cardiovascular training is so effective because it causes a physiological disturbance your body has to recover from, and the act of recovering is what is causing your body to burn significantly more calories during the following 24 to 48 hours. Because the intensity of your interval training is so important to its success, be sure to approach it with the same mentality as your strength training: make sure you're well rested, well nourished, well hydrated, and focused on working your hardest.

Following are some examples of effective high intensity cardio workouts. Always perform a 5 to 10 minute warm-up and dynamic stretch session to prevent sprains and strains.

30/20/10 Sprint Drills

Work at a very slow pace for 30 seconds, a challenging pace for 20 seconds, and then go all out for 10 seconds for a total cycle time of one minute. This is one 30/20/10 cycle. For a full workout, repeat for two to four sets of these cycles for a total of five minutes, resting for two-three minutes between sets. For example, a complete two-set workout will look like this:

- Begin with a 5 to 10 minute warm-up and dynamic stretching.
- Begin work sets with a 30 second interval at a slow pace. Increase to a challenging pace for 20 seconds. Increase to an all out pace for 10 seconds. Immediately drop to your slowest pace for the next cycle.
- Repeat the above 30/20/10 cycle four more times for a total of five work sets.
- Rest completely for two to three minutes.
- Repeat the 30/20/10 cycle five times as above.
- Complete the workout with some light cardio and static stretching as needed.

Hill Sprints

Choose a fairly steep hill that you can sprint up in 10 to 30 seconds at maximal effort. Perform 6 to 8 sets of hill sprints, walking back down to the starting point giving yourself 1 to 2 minutes to recover (including walking to the bottom) between sets.

Short Distance Sprints

Choose a set distance of flat, level ground (ideally a field or track) that you can cover in about 20 seconds at maximal effort. Sprint the chosen distance for 8 to 12 sets, giving yourself 40 seconds to recover between sets.

Long Distance Sprints

Choose a set distance that you can cover in about one minute at maximal effort. Sprint the chosen distance for 6 to 8 sets, giving yourself two to three minutes to recover between sets.

Stationary Bike Sprints

On a stationary bike, choose a challenging resistance that still allows you to reach a maximum cadence and perform intervals of 20 seconds at maximum speed, recovering for 40 seconds at an easy pace. Repeat for 8 to 12 total sets. Once this becomes easy, intervals can be progressed to 30 seconds at maximum effort and 30 seconds recovery.

Tabata Sets

One of the fastest and most brutal HIIT programs available is a Tabata interval, created by a Japanese Olympic speed skating coach. To perform Tabata sets, choose a challenging exercise such as a rowing machine, battle ropes, jump rope, prowler sled, etc, and perform intervals of 20 seconds at maximum intensity, resting for ONLY 10 seconds between intervals. Repeat eight times for a total of four minutes. If desired, rest completely for 2 to 3 minutes and repeat for up to three additional Tabata sets on different exercises, for a total of 4 four-minute sets with 2 to 3 minutes rest between each.

Swimming Sprints

This is Derek's favorite because they engage the upper body as well as the lower body and are zero impact, making them excellent for reducing and recovering from injuries. Warm up by swimming 8 to 10 laps (400-500 meters), then perform intervals of one lap (50 meters) maximal effort and one lap recovery for 6 to 8 sets, or one length (25 meters) maximal effort and one length recovery for 8 to 10 sets.

Car/Sled Sprints

If you have access to a prowler sled they are a fantastic conditioning and strength building tool and, if not, a car in neutral works nearly as well! Just be sure to turn the car off during your sprints so you aren't inhaling exhaust, then get back in and drive it back to the starting point during your rest intervals. Find an open area such as a large empty parking lot and, after your warm up, push the sled/car with maximal effort over a set distance that takes approximately 20 seconds to cover. Rest one minute and repeat for 6 to 10 sets.

Chapter 3: Nutrition Strategies

There are two major objectives in every off-season: to build as much muscle as possible with minimal fat gain and to stimulate your metabolism. It is important that your diet addresses both of these goals or your progress will not be optimal. Fortunately, it is possible to plan your diet with both of these goals in mind.

There are four macronutrients: protein, carbohydrates, fats, and fiber. Three of these are the source of all your dietary calories. Bodybuilders as a group pay very close attention to how much of each macronutrient they take in, in addition to total calories, to maximize their goals. Contrary to popular opinion, all calories are not created equal, which is why paying attention to macronutrients is important and why a diet composed of whole plant foods, as opposed to the same amount of calories from any other kind of food, can yield such amazing health outcomes.

Protein

In addition to providing calories (4 cal/gram), protein is also a structural molecule that builds tissues such as muscle. Protein intake can help meet the goal of metabolic stimulation as well, to some extent. Protein takes more energy to digest than any other macronutrient, which means that your body is burning calories just to break down your food. This is why there is so much emphasis on getting 'enough' for bodybuilders. Many assume that if they can just cram in enough protein, the muscles will follow. It's not that simple! While eating the right amount of protein at the right time can stimulate muscle building (protein synthesis), overconsumption can be detrimental. It puts a burden on your liver and kidneys as it gets removed from the body and the extra calories you're taking in could be stored as fat. These risks are far less of an issue when consuming plant proteins, but should still be kept in mind. According to the American College of Sports Medicine, strength and power athletes will optimize their performance by consuming 1.6 to 1.8 grams of protein per kilogram of bodyweight each day (which comes out to about 0.8 grams per pound of weight), about half of what is commonly recommended! So why is more protein being recommended everywhere you look? Is more really better?

A study entitled "Effect of Protein Intake on Strength, Body Composition and Endocrine Changes in Strength/Power Athletes" published in the December 2006 issue of the *Journal of the International Society of Sports Nutrition* set out to test if protein above these recommendations was, in fact, better. They placed 23 collegiate strength/power athletes on a diet below, at, or above the ACSM recommended protein intakes while being the same in total calories and had them follow a 12 week strength training program. At the end of the program they tested each athlete's improvements in strength and lean body mass, and guess what they found? There was no significant difference between any of the groups in any of these measures. All 23 participants improved in strength and body composition, and while there were slight differences in each group amounting to a slightly better result in the higher protein groups, it was not statistically significant and so was just as likely due to random chance as to the variables tested.

So, what is the ideal amount of protein then? Like anything else, this varies from person to person, but based on the latest research as well our own experience, we recommend taking in 1.6 grams of protein per kilogram of body weight (1.6 g/kg, or 0.75g/lb) as a minimum and 2.2 g/kg (or 1.0g/lb) as a maximum yields excellent results while avoiding the physical stress of overconsumption.

This is enough to ensure that if your body needs to use some protein for fuel it will come from food rather than your existing muscle, yet not so much that will become a threat to your body as the excess is excreted or crowd out other nutrients that could be in your diet. Too much concern over protein is especially unnecessary during the off-season because you are taking in a calorie surplus, making it much more likely that the protein you consume will be used to build new tissue (or get stored as fat) and much less likely to be burned as fuel.

Please remember that the maximum recommendations are for hard-training athletes. A typical sedentary individual should not consume any more than the minimum recommendations above, simply because there is no physiological need for it, making any extra protein consumed nothing but an additional calorie burden. It's far better to get extra calories from produce which will certainly not be stored as fat and will provide additional antioxidants and micronutrients besides!

Carbohydrates

As an herbivore, you probably already know that carbohydrates are extremely important for your well-being and long-term health. As a bodybuilder they are just as vital. Carbohydrate sources should make up the majority of your diet, especially in the off-season, as they are essential for meeting your goals.

Carbohydrates are important in muscle-building for two reasons: they fuel intense training more effectively than other calorie sources and when you are getting enough calories from carbohydrates your body is virtually guaranteed not to break down protein, in the form of your existing muscles, for energy. This means that almost all of the protein you eat is available for generating new muscle tissue.

Carbohydrates are also essential for stimulating your metabolism. While they don't require as much energy to digest as proteins do, they do require more energy to digest than fat and, in addition, have the greatest thermic effect of any calorie source (burning energy as body heat). By slowly adding calories, especially carbohydrates, to your diet in the off-season you can easily increase your basal metabolic rate by as much as 100%. Making this effort initially will allow you to start your dieting later with a racing metabolism and plenty of calories available to cut out without leaving you starving.

Of course, the carbohydrate sources we're referring to here are whole foods and complex starches like oats, quinoa, brown rice, and sweet potatoes. Fruits are a healthy addition to your diet as well, but the majority of your carbohydrates should come from complex starches.

For macronutrient tracking purposes, carbohydrates should make up a minimum of 50% of your calories during the off-season but limiting them to a strict amount in grams generally isn't recommended. Once you have your target protein and fat intake amounts determined, you could adjust your target carbohydrate intake to reach your desired calorie intake and when you periodically raise your calories over the course of the off-season these additional calories should come from carbohydrate sources.

Fat

Dietary fat is the third source of calories in your diet and, while fat is important for many physiological functions, it is also important to keep your intake at a fairly low level in order to avoid excess body fat gain. This is because dietary fat has by far the *most* concentrated calories at 9 per gram yet takes the *least* amount of energy to both digest and store as body fat.

However, dietary fat is extremely important for making gains and recovering during the off-season. It regulates hormone production and inflammation within the body, both of which are closely tied to recovery from exercise and subsequent supercompensation. The primary hormone fat effects is one that bodybuilders are concerned with: testosterone. Testosterone is a male sex hormone but is produced by both sexes and having optimal levels will increase strength and muscle gain after training, decrease recovery time, and speed the metabolism to enhance fat burning.

The optimal amount of dietary fat to consume during the off-season is roughly 0.3 to 0.5 grams per pound of body weight, which is about 20% of total calories. This is a range, and where you fall will depend on your body type, as endomorphs will want to stay at the lower end while ectomorphs can afford to stay at the higher end of the range. This level of fat intake has been shown to maximize testosterone production. Consume less than around 20% and you run the risk of hindering your gains; consume much more than this and you will increase your fat gains, which will be counterproductive.

Healthy sources of fat to include in your diet are whole plant foods such as nuts, seeds, olives, and avocados, but remember that even when you are avoiding these high fat foods (such as during the dieting phase of your contest preparation) all healthy plant foods contain some fat so you will still be getting all that you need. "Getting enough fat" is a common, and unnecessary, concern on a vegan diet, and we often have to break clients of the habit of snacking on nuts and oils to meet a perceived need to do so. Even oats contain a significant amount of fat, for example, and it is very easy to reach that 20% range with no added oils and even minimal high fat plant foods like avocados.

What About Omega-3 Fatty Acids?

The type of fat that you take in - saturated, monounsaturated, or polyunsaturated - does have health consequences. Saturated fats in general should be avoided, so don't be misled by health claims made about coconut and palm oils, while a fat you *should* make sure you're eating on a daily basis is omega-3s. Omega-3 fatty acids are polyunsaturated fats with essential roles throughout the body such as reducing inflammation, and eating a diet with higher concentrations has been shown to decrease the risk of a whole host of chronic degenerative diseases. This is especially important for a hard training bodybuilder because omega-3s will aid muscle recovery and growth and they are something you may need to go out of your way to get enough of. Most whole food plant sources like nuts, seeds and avocados have some omega-3s, but, if you are concerned about getting enough, make flax seeds, chia seeds, hemp, and walnuts your fat sources and you will get all you need!

Sample Off-Season Meal Plans

Now we come to the million-dollar question: what do you actually *eat*? Even among the vegan bodybuilding community, a wide spectrum of eating styles is represented, from supplement-laden, to raw, to vegan Paleo. Our recommendation is to consume primarily whole plant foods with minimal supplementation. Following are two examples of what such a bodybuilding menu might look like. We also include menus from our own meal plans in the appendix. All of the menus, recipes, and templates provided in this book are applicable to both genders and any division as long as you tailor the portions to meet *your* calorie, protein, carbohydrate, and fat intake targets. You'll also notice the different timing of meals depending on the time of day workouts are scheduled. Some people prefer to work out first thing in the morning on an empty stomach (this is our preferred method) and others like to snack on some fruit beforehand for increased energy, while still others work out in the afternoons as their schedule allows. Whatever the case may be, make sure you get a quick post-workout meal afterward, with or without protein powders.

Menu #1

Pre-Workout:
Banana
Post-Workout:
Protein Shake with
Full Serving Vegan Protein Powder
Soy Milk
Breakfast:
Oatmeal
Fresh Blueberries
Snack:
Derek's "Bean Shake" with:
Banana
Cannellini Beans
Oatmeal
Spinach
Pumpkin Seeds
Frozen Strawberries
Half Serving Vegan Protein Powder
Lunch:
Green Salad
Red Lentil Soup
Baked Sweet Potato
Snack:
Derek's "Bean Shake"
Dinner:
Green Salad
Brown Rice Pasta
Lentil and Vegetable Tomato Sauce
Steamed Leafy Greens

Menu #2

Breakfast:
Smoothie with:

Banana
Dates
Frozen Spinach
Frozen Berries
Pre-Workout:
Dates
Post-Workout:
Smoothie with:
Silken Tofu
Frozen Mango
Kale
Snack:
Kiwi
Lunch:
Chickpea Salad
Steamed Potatoes
Steamed Green Beans
Snack:
Derek's "Bean Shake" with
Banana
Cannellini Beans
Spinach
Pumpkin Seeds
Frozen Strawberries
Dinner:
Quinoa Tabouli
Broccoli Soup

Derek's "Bean Shake" Template

One of the most popular articles we've shared on our website is Derek's recipe for a vegan weight-gainer shake, or as it has come to be known, the bean shake. What makes this shake in all its variations special is that it combines healthy whole plant foods such as beans and greens in a convenient form that makes it easy to get them in throughout the day, causing any gains to come from quality, nutrient-dense food. These shakes have helped Derek gain 20 pounds of lean muscle mass and have worked similar magic for Marcella and countless clients; in fact, "bean shake" has become part of the lexicon of the vegan bodybuilding community! The best part is that the recipe can also easily be tailored to your needs, whether you are trying to gain muscle or lose body fat. What follows is a blueprint. You need not, and should not, use every possible ingredient listed. Instead, choose according to your preferences and tolerances among the foods listed with your goals in mind. For example, someone who has a very difficult time gaining weight will need to go heavy on the calorie-dense starches and fats in the off-season, while someone who still has body fat to lose pre-contest will entirely avoid high fat additions.

You will need:

- A powerful blender, such as a Vitamix
- Several large smoothie containers
- Bulk quantities of the ingredients you decide to use for your shakes.

Choose from the ingredients listed below.

Protein Sources

- White beans: Cannellini, Great Northern, or navy beans have the mildest flavor and best texture.
- Tofu: Choose a soft or silken variety for a creamy texture.
- Peas: They have a sweet flavor.
- Protein Supplements (optional): For those of you who choose to use protein supplements, these serve as an easy source of extra protein and also as a flavor enhancer. Just be sure to include some whole food protein also so you don't miss out on any nutrition

Carbohydrates

- Fruits: Bananas and berries are a standard choice, but everything aside from citrus will work well.
- Grains: Oatmeal or oat bran (raw), quinoa (cooked), brown rice (cooked), grits (cooked) can all add extra calories and nutrition
- Starchy vegetables: Carrots (raw) or sweet potatoes (cooked) can also add a lot of nutrition and more calories

Fats (Avoid If Reducing Body Fat)

- Seeds: Any will work, but a favorite choice is raw hulled pumpkin seeds because they have a great amino acid profile and a lot of minerals. Flax or chia seeds are a good choice as well for omega-3 fatty acids.
- Nut butters
- Avocado
- Coconut: We don't recommend using coconut oil because it is a processed, concentrated fat, but raw coconut flesh would be a good flavor enhancer.

Other Additions

- Vegetables: Maximize these to get in extra nutrition. We add heaps of frozen spinach, which doesn't affect the flavor and is extremely nutritious. There are many other great options; the more the better!
- Flavor Enhancers: Tasty additions include fruit, coconut water, flavored protein powder, non-dairy milks or yogurt (which also serve as protein sources, but are processed), nut butters, sweeteners such as fruit juice or maple syrup, spices such as cinnamon or nutmeg, cocoa powder, and coconut. Keep in mind that some of these are not fat-loss friendly.

The amounts of each ingredient are based entirely on your goals and taste preferences. Here is a version that Derek has used extensively:

Derek's Off-Season Bean Shake
Makes 2 servings

2 Ripe Bananas

1 Cup Oats

2 Cups Soymilk

3 Cups Great Northern Beans

1/4 Cup Pumpkin Seeds

1 cup Frozen Strawberries

1 cup Frozen Spinach

1 Scoop Vegan Protein Powder

Water to desired thickness

Approximate Totals per Serving: 860 calories, 55 g protein, 135 g carbs, 15 g fat (25/60/15 macronutrient ratio)

And, to demonstrate the variation possible according to goals and personal statistics, here is Marcella's stripped-down, low fat version:

Marcella's Pre-Contest Bean Shake
Makes 2 servings

½ Ripe Banana

1 Cup Soymilk

½ Cup Cannellini Beans

½ Scoop Vegan Protein Powder

Water to desired thickness

Approximate Totals per Serving: 301 calories, 27 g protein, 40 g carbs, 5 g fat (35/50/15 macronutrient ratio)

Guide to Cheat Meals

Cheat meals: the off-season's most popular topic! As mentioned previously, there is a commonly held belief that a competitor should regularly binge on junk food to help them make the gains in strength and mass they seek, and we know now that this is not optimal because it can lead to excess fat gain and can hinder performance. However, there are some physical and psychological benefits to an occasional 'treat' meal.

Consuming richer and more concentrated calories than you are accustomed to will cause your body to release two important hormones in abundant supply: insulin and leptin. Insulin pulls nutrients from your bloodstream into your muscle cells, giving them ample fuel to recover and grow. When you eat food that is richer and a more concentrated calorie source than you are used to, the amount of insulin you release after the meal is much higher than usual, which immediately halts muscle breakdown and simultaneously engorges the muscle cells with calories and nutrients.

Leptin is one of the most important hormones for regulating fat burning. It increases your BMR (basal metabolic rate), increases your use of body fat for energy, and can decrease your appetite. After a cheat meal your body releases an abundance of leptin, which stimulates your metabolism and, as long as you immediately return to eating clean, stimulates improved fat burning.

Another benefit of scheduled cheat meals is that for some they make eating a strict diet the majority of the time easier to handle! Of course, many people are content to eat clean whole foods all of the time but for those who struggle, the cheat meal can help break up the monotony and prevent discouragement. A regularly scheduled meal out helps people in this situation stay focused on reaping the benefits of eating almost all healthy whole foods while still being able to look forward to favorite foods and social meals with friends. And, of course, remember that cheat meals are still always vegan.

It's important to note that the above benefits of cheat meals only apply if the schedule is rigorously adhered to and they are an infrequent occurrence of no more than one or two times a week. Eating rich meals at widely spaced intervals ensures that your body will be sensitive enough to reap the hormonal benefits of the unusually rich food, whereas eating these foods regularly, even in small amounts tailored to your macros, can limit the shock to your system and corresponding metabolism jumpstart, increase your insulin resistance, and make your normal healthy diet seem far less desirable.

Scheduling Your Cheat Meals

You can schedule your cheat meal during the week however you like, as long as you don't indulge in them too often. However, there *are* some times at which you can reap even greater benefits from a cheat meal:

- **After training a stubborn body part.** Everyone has a muscle group or two that lags behind the rest of their body. The anabolic nature of a cheat meal can help stimulate a weak body part.

- **On leg day, after your workout.** It's no secret that legs are the most demanding and strenuous muscle group to train. These are the biggest, strongest muscles in your body with the greatest stamina. They require the most oxygen and calories to train and training them elicits the greatest anabolic response post-training. This puts your body in an excellent position to use extra calories from rich foods.
- **On a high intensity cardio day, after your workout.** Performing high intensity cardio, such as track sprints, has a similar effect on your body as a leg training workout, making it another excellent time to schedule some excess calories.

Choosing Your Cheat Meals Wisely

Yes, a cheat meal is your opportunity to eat some of those less-than-healthy foods you've been avoiding on your normal diet, but rather than engaging in an eating free-for-all, stick to these guidelines:

- You do want extra calories, but more is not better. Rather than hitting seconds and thirds at the all-you-can-eat buffet, go out to your favorite restaurant and order a salad, get an appetizer, an entree, and share a dessert with a friend. This way you'll be getting a big bump in calories and having a decadent meal, but portions will still be controlled to some extent.
- In terms of metabolic boost, carbs are king. The primary hormone you want to increase with a cheat meal is leptin, and this hormone responds almost exclusively to your carbohydrate intake. Great choices for cheats are everyone's favorite carb-loading foods like pizza, pasta, sandwiches, and pastries.
- Since carbohydrates are your target food, try to go easy on your fat intake to avoid overshooting your metabolic boost with too many calories. Stay away from fried foods, and high-fat entrees and desserts. Splitting a slice of vegan pie after a reasonable meal won't wreck you, but eating a vegan cheeseburger with fries and a vegan ice cream sundae might.
- If you feel you went a little too far with your cheat meal, go ahead and reduce calories the next day by 10% or add 30 to 45 minutes of extra steady-state cardio and you should be fine!

Supplements

No text on bodybuilding would be complete without at least a brief discussion of supplements. We will review some that are commonly consumed here, but let us first state that we do not believe that supplements are necessary to be successful as a bodybuilder. There is ample research showing that some supplements help improve performance or body composition, but never feel that you must take them in order to achieve your goals in this or any other sport. The foundation of your success will always be your nutrition, training and recovery. Supplements may bring you a few extra percent of improvement, but remember that they are a *supplement* to your nutrition and training regimen, not the core of it.

There are several supplements that are commonly used and may be effective, so we'd like to discuss them here.

Protein

The most widely used class of supplements by far are protein powders. A common mistake made by new vegans is an overreliance on protein powders to hit the daily intake they think they need. A protein supplement is an easy and convenient way to increase the protein concentration in your diet without increasing calories too much, and has been shown to aid in muscle recovery and growth, but getting too much protein from supplements rather than whole foods means you are missing out on a lot of nutrition found only in whole food. Our rule of thumb, if you choose to supplement with protein powder, is to keep supplemented protein under 20% of total protein intake (and preferably closer to 10%). This will ensure that you are getting the bulk of your protein from healthy, nutrient dense sources like green vegetables, legumes and whole grains.

When choosing a brand of protein, some things to look for are minimal processing, a combination of multiple sources of plant proteins, and organic or raw ingredients. This will ensure that the product is as nutritious as possible, has a broad spectrum of amino acids, and will have the least possible industrial contaminants. Some brands we recommend are PlantFusion, SunWarrior, and Vega.

Creatine

Creatine is a supplement that is nearly as widely used and researched as protein. Its purported benefits are increased strength and strength endurance (more reps with a heavy weight), and there is substantial evidence showing its effectiveness in this regard. It functions by being stored within muscle cells (where it also naturally occurs) as a source of fuel for very high intensity activities, and by supplementing the diet with it we are able to increase the amount stored within our muscle cell and increase our ability to work at a high intensity.

Creatine comes in many forms, with the most common being creatine monohydrate. Our recommendation, if you choose to supplement, is creatine monohydrate for low cost or, for a slightly higher price, Kre-Alkalyn. Kre-Alkalyn has personally yielded the most consistent results, and has the advantages of not requiring loading or cycling, not causing water retention, and a lower dosage than other forms.

BCAAs

Branched Chain Amino Acids (Leucine, Isoleucine and Valine) are essential amino acids found in protein, and are the biochemically active compounds which allow protein to trigger new muscle synthesis independent of exercise by stimulating the biochemical pathway mTOR. Of the three, Leucine is the most important, and even just adding leucine to various plant proteins such as wheat gluten has been shown to make them even more anabolic (muscle building) than whey protein from cow's milk. BCAA supplementation during training, especially when under a caloric deficit, had been shown to improve gains in muscle mass and reduce muscle loss, but new research has also shown the the mTOR biochemical pathway may be linked to disease later in life, and might even reduce longevity. As with all supplements, do your homework and make an informed decision based on your personal goals.

Caffeine

Since it is so widely consumed in the form of coffee, tea, and soda, caffeine is rarely considered a supplement, but it does have measurable and consistent effects on performance and body composition, and therefore makes its way into many supplement cocktails. Caffeine is a stimulant of the central nervous system, and when taken before exercise has been shown to increase motivation, improve performance in both strength and endurance, and aid in body fat loss through increasing caloric expenditure. That's a pretty long list of 'pros'. The cons are that caffeine is an instant advance on your energy of the next 24 hours and will therefore leave you feeling less energetic and alert once it wears off. Consistently taking caffeine in any form will raise your tolerance and can easily lead to dependence and chronic fatigue. If you choose to supplement with it in any form, take the minimum amount you can for the desired effect, and make sure you have one or more days per week where you don't have any at all so that your tolerance doesn't increase.

Pre-Workout Supplement Cocktails

A whole class of supplements marketed as pre-workouts claim to enhance your motivation, energy, strength, performance, muscle pumps, and endurance. While many of them do at least some of what they claim to, they generally have 'proprietary blends' of ingredients, which could include almost anything. If we are to consider supplements in general as risky and likely not good for long-term health, a cocktail of mystery chemicals should raise some serious concerns. If a company you trust provides a pre-workout without any proprietary blends and you'd like to try it out, here are some components they may contain and why:

- A stimulant, usually caffeine, for enhanced energy, motivation, and work capacity
- Some form of creatine for enhanced strength and strength endurance
- A nitric oxide boosting compound to increase blood flow to working muscle and aid in achieving a 'pump' which is usually L-Arginine, L-Carnitine, or Agmatine Sulfate
- Amino acids such as glutamine or BCAAs
- Added antioxidants, herbal supplements, or extracts

Testosterone Boosters

As a class of supplements, T-Boosters have the most diverse and inconsistent ingredients out there, many of which are unsupported by scientific evidence and often hidden within a proprietary blend. As with pre-workouts, this should be a red flag. These supplements may be effective however, and claim to work by increasing the body's natural production of testosterone while also reducing production of estrogen and cortisol, two hormones that can negatively impact your physique. Shifting your hormones in this way will increase strength, muscle mass, and recovery rate while also reducing body fat. If you're interested in trying a test-booster, look for a reputable brand with all ingredients listed and no proprietary blends, and be sure to cycle it as directed on the label (usually on for 4 to 8 weeks and off for 4 weeks) to maintain your natural production of testosterone and prevent dependence. This is generally a class of supplements targeted to males, and will be most effective in men over thirty years old or men with naturally low testosterone because these individuals will see the largest relative increase in free testosterone.

Fat Burners

Fat burners are another class of supplements with a very wide spectrum of possible ingredients. Much like pre-workouts and testosterone boosters, proceed with caution and avoid anything with a proprietary blend. Fat burners are marketed to assist in body fat loss by increasing energy and caloric expenditure while decreasing appetite. Common ingredients are stimulants such as caffeine and herbal supplements like green coffee extract. While some fat burner cocktails do increase the rate of body fat loss, we believe them to be an unnecessary risk, and have never used them ourselves or with clients.

Chapter 4: Choosing a Contest

When planning your off-season goals and programming it can be very helpful to have a contest chosen so that you have a precise time frame in mind. There are several things to consider as you compare potential events: location, size, organization, and time of year.

The location of your contest is very important because it coul increase your competition expenses in the form of airfare, transportation, missed work, meals out and more. It can also impact your overall experience. Traveling a long distance can also affect the amount of support from friends and family you will have, and the condition in which you will arrive. Does travel cause you to bloat and retain water, for example? If so you may want to fly in a couple of days early!

The size of the city hosting the contest will also give you an idea of the size of the show, as a larger city usually means more competitors and a higher overall level of competition. A small town, on the other hand, will have fewer competitors and fewer veterans among them.

Different bodybuilding organizations hold contests in different regions and also differ in size and level of prestige. A larger and more prestigious organization will have a bigger budget and stage a better event...and will attract the stiffest competition. The largest amateur organizations are currently the National Physique Committee (NPC), which does not drug test its athletes, and the International Natural Bodybuilding Federation (INBF), which does test its athletes. Competing in a non drug-tested event means that you may be competing against athletes on steroids or other drugs, so keep that in mind. Each of these amateur organizations affiliate with very competitive pro organizations such as the IFBB, WNBF, or the IFPA, which is another very competitive drug-tested organization with 8 affiliated amateur organizations. So if a contest you're interested in is a pro-qualifying show with one these groups, prepare for a tough battle!

A comprehensive schedule of natural bodybuilding events can be found at www.naturalbodybuildingevents.com, including all natural bodybuilding organizations and events around the world, making it an excellent resource for choosing a contest by either date, organization, or location. Pro-qualifying events will be indicated with a (PQ) next to the event title or within the description. Pro-Qualifying events allow division overall winners, for example, the overall winner in open men's bodybuilding, to obtain a pro card and move on to compete within the affiliated pro organization for cash prizes. Winning a pro qualifying event does not mean that you have to compete as a professional, but if you choose to you will no longer be eligible to compete within that amateur division, and, of course, the pro contests you move on to compete in will be much more competitive.

Time of year can also be a deciding factor. The bodybuilding season runs from March to November with most of the largest and most competitive shows taking place toward the end of the season. Keeping in mind your projected off-season length and the three to five months needed to diet and get into show condition, the time you choose to compete can end up having a big impact on how easy your prep is. For example, are you willing to be on a strict diet throughout the holiday season? Will you have an easier time doing lots of cardio while you are hungry and grumpy in beautiful spring weather, or will you hold up better in a cold gym in the dead of winter? These considerations can make a world of difference in how enjoyable your experience is, so take the time to give it some careful thought before you begin!

Photo by Josh Avery

Section 2: Pre-Contest

The pre-contest phase is the time period when a bodybuilder shifts gears in preparation for an upcoming show. Whereas the off-season has the objectives of gaining maximum muscle mass, minimal fat mass, and stimulating the metabolism, the pre-contest period has the major focus of shedding body fat while preserving muscle mass and the secondary goal of doing everything possible to improve your showing on stage. This phase is also commonly referred to as the "cutting" phase.

Included in the following chapters are examples of how nutrition, weight training, and cardio exercise are progressed throughout this phase to keep getting results. These sample progressions worked for a client seeking to go from 180 pounds to a 165-pound contest weight. Similar progressions can work for anyone; the volume of training, the amount of calories consumed, and the amount of cardio do not depend on gender or even division but instead depend entirely on goals. All that is required is to calculate the numbers that fit your goals, your current state, and your targets to apply these same progressions in your contest planning!

Chapter 5: Calculating a Time Frame

So you've had a productive off-season, gained some solid lean muscle, maintained a healthy level of body fat, and you have a contest picked out. Assuming that you've allowed yourself ample time for the off-season and that the contest is still several months away, you need to decide when to begin your diet and get into 'pre-contest' mode.

The amount of time each competitor needs to get into stage shape will vary widely based on age, gender, metabolism, initial amount of body fat, and previous contest experience, but here are some general guidelines.

Slower is always better. If you've taken your time adding muscle mass and eating plenty of calories from healthy whole foods your metabolism should be humming along at a fast pace and your body should be primed to shed body fat. The last thing you want to do at this point is go on a crash diet, cutting too many calories over too short a period of time, to meet an impossibly near deadline and undo all of the hard work of the months before. Given that you would be starting from a metabolic high point you would be able to shed fat very quickly with deep calorie cuts, but doing so would also shed much more of your hard-earned muscle mass than necessary and dramatically slow your metabolism in the process, making post-contest fat gain all too likely. Steep drops in your caloric intake will also reduce your performance in the gym and slow your recovery after training, leaving you weak and tired and again causing you to shed still more muscle.

Give yourself 16 weeks, minimum, to prepare. Since we know that slower is better when it comes to fat loss, it makes sense that we should have a minimum time frame for getting ready to compete.

Every athlete is different and some can certainly get ready in as little as 10 weeks but, for inexperienced competitors or those who have just added mass, it's a good idea to play it safe and give yourself a large buffer. Derek has made the mistake of allowing too little time to diet and the result was that he took the stage with too much body fat and placed poorly in a show that should have been an easy win. In natural bodybuilding competitions, winners are chosen by conditioning (low body fat) over all other attributes so it makes sense to ensure that you will be at your leanest! In 16 weeks almost anyone with a healthy low level of body fat eating ample clean calories can get into excellent condition with no crash dieting, making this a perfect minimum time frame.

Use the amount of fat you have to lose to set a time frame to prepare. In previous chapters we learned how to calculate our lean body mass and our total pounds of body fat. We also supplied an approximate guide to target body fat levels for different divisions. Using this information you can calculate your: a) current pounds of body fat and b) pounds of body fat you will have in your target contest condition, keeping your lean mass constant. If you subtract b) from a) you'll have the total pounds of fat you need to lose. In our goal setting chapter we discussed that an ideal rate of fat loss that minimizes muscle loss is one to two pounds per week. Unless you have more than 20 pounds of fat to lose, slower is better, so shoot for about one pound of fat loss per week and use your target fat loss total to determine the length of your diet. If you have more than 20 pounds of fat to lose, use the slowest rate of loss you can to confine your diet to 24 weeks or less - ideally keeping your loss rate at or below 2 pounds per week. A simple calculation will demonstrate that these guidelines are impossible if you have 50 or more pounds to lose. If that is the case, we strongly suggest taking 6 to 12 months to build more muscle and improve your body composition before committing to a contest diet.

Weekly Goals and Assessments

Now that you've calculated the total weight you must lose and, using the guidelines of the previous chapter, the length of time your diet will be, it's time to set weekly goals. We strongly advise you to set your target end date one to two weeks before your contest so that you have a safety buffer for any plateaus and so that you can focus all of your efforts on peaking in the final week. With this in mind, create a chart (we use an Excel spreadsheet) filled in with your target body fat and weight for each week of your diet. These can be calculated using the program if you're Excel-savvy, or manually as follows: Divide both your total pounds of fat to lose and your percentage of body fat to lose by the number of weeks of your diet. This gives you a weekly expected change to subtract from the previous week to get the next week's projected weight and body fat. For example, let's say you are currently 12% fat and have a target of 6% that you plan to achieve in 12 weeks, giving you 6% to lose. Six percent divided by 12 gives you a projected loss of ½% per week. Let's also say you weigh 215 pounds and hope to weigh 200 by your contest date, giving you 15 pounds to lose. This gives you a projected loss of 1.25 pounds per week. Based on these numbers, your chart might look like this:

End of Week	Projected % Body Fat	Actual % Body Fat	Projected Weight	Actual Weight
1	11.5		213.75	
2	11		212.5	
3	10.5		211.25	
4	10		210	
5	9.5		208.75	
6	9		207.5	
7	8.5		206.25	
8	8		205	
9	7.5		203.75	
10	7		202.5	
11	6.5		201.25	
12	6		200	

Set one day each week as your assessment day on which you weigh yourself and calculate your body fat percentage, giving you actual numbers to compare to your weekly goals. This weekly check-in is extremely important to catch any plateaus or steep drops in time to make adjustments and to keep you accountable and motivated. We also strongly suggest you take a video or still shots of your posing every week on assessment day so you can get a visual of your progress. This will not only help you keep track of your current progression, it will give you reference points of what you can expect to look like at different weights and body fat levels for future contest planning.

It's important to keep in mind that most biological processes don't happen in a linear fashion, and this includes the changes you hope to see in your body. As long as you are approximately keeping pace with your targets there is no need to panic, but if you are stuck for two to three weeks it is time to progress either your diet or your cardio, or both. Since you are trying to shed fat slowly and maintain your metabolic rate as much as possible, the simplest adjustment is to reduce daily caloric intake by about 100 to 200 calories. Try not to drop your calories more often than once every week, and by no more than 200 calories, however. Steep drops will slow your metabolism. This is a general overview; a detailed progression is outlined below.

Chapter 6: Progressions to Meet Your Weekly Goals

Nutrition Progressions

Begin your diet. Reduce or, better yet, eliminate all processed foods, especially refined carbohydrates such as flour products. You may also reduce your daily calorie intake by 100 to 200 calories at this point. Cheat meals are not advised, but one every 10 to 14 days will not cause too much harm.

When weight loss slows, reduce daily calories by another 100 to 200, preferably from fat and then carbohydrates. When reducing carbohydrates, first reduce those that are high glycemic such as tropical fruits and white potatoes. Repeat this calorie reduction whenever weight loss is slowed or stopped for two to three weeks.

Carry on as above for as long as possible, cutting calories as infrequently as you can. If your fat loss remains stalled after a reduction or if you've fallen behind your target and need to make up ground it's time to start cycling your carbohydrates and calories.

Carb Cycling

1. Increase your daily protein intake above 1 gram per pound of body weight to preserve muscle mass and drop your daily calories approximately 300 to 400 calories below what you are currently consuming to maintain your weight. To keep your protein percentage high you will have to start viewing legumes as a starch and increase foods such as tofu, tempeh, and seitan while reducing fruits and starches. Fat intake should already

be very low at this point, but if fats make up more than 20% of your daily calories reduce them as well. Your macronutrient breakdown will now likely be around 40/40/20 or 50/30/20 (Protein/Carbohydrate/Fat) unless you were still consuming a lot of carbohydrates up to this point. Ideally, your target daily calories should be no less than 60% of your maintenance calories when you started your diet. The closer to your starting point you are, the higher your metabolic rate.

2. Starting with the first day you begin carb cycling, consume a 'refeed' day every seven days (once per week). On refeed day, increase your calories to about 50% above your maintenance level (not your new dieting amount) making the majority of the increase from carbohydrates. The objective of a refeed day is to stimulate your metabolism so the lower caloric intake of your diet doesn't slow it down as quickly and you can keep losing fat. Foods you'd normally avoid are permissible on these days (think bread, pasta, cereal, bagels, muffins, low fat pizza). You should still get in healthy whole food carbohydrates such as whole grains, root vegetables, and fruit on these days as well. Be careful to keep your fat intake low, however, or the refeed days may do more harm than good.

3. Continue carb cycling at this level until progress stalls again, even for just one week. At this point, reduce your low days by another 100 to 200 calories and reduce your refeed days by 300 to 500 calories using the same guidelines as above. This should be sufficient to get things moving again but if you have another stalled week after the first, change your refeed day protocol. Increase your calories on that day back to initial levels and add more 'cheat' foods to provide a bigger metabolic stimulus; your metabolism may be getting stubborn. You may want to decrease your low days even further by 100 to 200 calories but this is optional unless you're weight loss is still slower than desired. Continue making reductions in the above fashion until peak week and include the extra-rich refeed days only as needed. If you're stalled near essential body fat levels (5% for men, 10% for women) you should include a second, smaller refeed day using only clean foods in the middle of the week as your body gradually becomes less

responsive to refeeds the leaner you get. For the smaller refeed, increase calories by 10 to 20 percent above your current maintenance level from whole food carbohydrates like oats, beans, brown rice, quinoa, and sweet or white potatoes. Some fruits are permissible as well.

Macronutrient Ratios

Your macronutrient ratio gives you a quick and comprehensive idea of where your diet is right now. The percentages of your calories that come from protein, carbohydrates, and fat can tell you much about why you may be having trouble reaching your goals. For example, a diet that is 40% fat from too many nuts and avocados quickly explains stubborn body fat that isn't responding to training. It's helpful information whenever you have a fitness goal, but when preparing for a competition it is critical. So how do you calculate it? Many competitors use free online tools, such as MyFitnessPal or apps such as Nutritionist to do so, and we also provide a free spreadsheet tool at our website, www.veganmuscleandfitness.com, for download. These will tell you where you are, but how do you calculate the grams from each macronutrient that you need to consume to stay near your target macronutrient ratio? Here's the nitty-gritty:

Multiply the amount of daily calories you want to consume by the decimal version of the percent of calories you'd like to come from a given macronutrient. For example, if in your new target ratio 50% of calories come from carbs, multiply by 0.5. This will give you the amount of your daily calories from carbs. Next, divide that number by the amount of calories per gram of the macronutrient, which for carbohydrates is 4 calories/gram.

So for example, if you consume 2,000 calories daily, multiply that by 0.5 to get 1,000 calories per day from carbohydrates, and then divide 1,000 calories by 4 calories per gram to arrive at a total of 250 grams of carbohydrates per day. Follow the same process for both protein and fats, except that fat has 9 calories per gram. So a 2,000 calorie a day diet with 20% of calories from fat will have 2,000 x 0.2 = 400 calories/9 calories per gram = 44 grams of fat.

Sample Nutrition Progressions

In this example, the 180-pound client sought to achieve a 165-pound contest weight. Your current statistics, goals, preferences, and, most importantly, your body's responses, will need to be taken into account when creating a plan. Each step following the starting point is determined based on the changes you've seen in your body following the previous step – this is why assessments are so critical to this process!

Off-season: Consumes about 3,000 calories per day with 200 grams of protein, 350 g carbs, and 90 g fat. Current weight is 180 lbs.

16 weeks out: Calories are kept the same, eating out is reduced to once per week (pretty clean), and all processed foods are eliminated. Weight has dropped from 180 lbs to 178 lbs.

14 weeks out: Reduces calories to 2,800 per day, with 200 grams protein, 325 g carbs, and 79 g fat. Weight has dropped from 178 lbs to 175 lbs, however weight loss has stalled after week 15 so another 200 calories per day, from carbs and fat, is cut.

11 weeks out: Calories are at 2,600 per day, with 200 grams protein, 300 g carbs, and 68 g fat. Weight has dropped from 175 lbs to 172 lbs. Again, weight loss has stopped so another 200 calories are cut.

9 weeks out: Calories are at 2,400 per day, with 210 grams protein, 265 g carbs, and 57 g fat. Weight has dropped from 172 lbs to 170 lbs and then stalled, so calories are dropped by 200 calories per day is cut.

6 weeks out: Weight loss has stalled and, with only six weeks remaining, we decided to implement carb cycling with one 'high' day and 6 'low' days. High days include 3,300 calories with 210 grams protein, 500 g carbs, and 50 g fat. Low days include 2,000 calories with 210 grams protein, 200 g carbs, and 42 g fat. Weight is now 167 lbs.

3 weeks out: With only two weeks left until peak week, we decided to prevent slowed progress by reducing calories by 10%. High days include 3,000 calories with 210 grams protein, 425 g carbs, and 50 g fat. Low days include 1,800 calories with 210 grams protein, 180 g carbs, and 38 g fat. Target weight of 165 lbs was reached one week early with extra time left over for peaking.

Training Progressions

Upon starting your diet, you should be doing two to three short and intense HIIT sessions per week. As you enter the pre-contest phase, your nutrition program will be the primary driver of your fat loss as you follow the outline provided in the previous chapter. Ideally, if your metabolic rate has improved enough during your off-season, simply making minor adjustments in your diet should be enough. If you begin to struggle to keep pace with your weekly goals, however, the following cardio progression should be implemented.

1. In addition to your current two to three HIIT sessions per week, add one 30-minute session at a steady rate, preferably fasted or after a weightlifting workout. The best options for steady cardio are a bike or step mill. Rowers can also be used if you feel they do not interfere with your training. Walking is a popular option, but has been shown to be less effective.
2. If your rate of fat loss slows further you can add an additional HIIT session up to a maximum of four per week. Be sure to separate your HIIT cardio from your workouts by several hours whenever possible so that you have optimal energy for both. Remember that HIIT workouts should never last longer than 25 minutes, including warm-up, to ensure that intensity and recovery are maximized.
3. Once you have reached four HIIT per week, when progress slows further you may add additional 30-minute steady sessions of cardio as necessary. Avoid doing cardio on leg days, as this workout requires the most recovery. Optimal times to schedule cardio are after training or fasted in the morning but you can fit them in whenever it works for you. Ideally no more than six total cardio workouts will be needed

during one week but, if you are lagging behind your goals, more 30 minute sessions can be added as second daily sessions; for example, one before breakfast and one before dinner.

4. As a last resort, the duration of either your steady or HIIT cardio workouts can be increased to get more in during the week. HIIT can be increased up to 35 minutes, including warm-up, and steady state can be increased to 45-minute sessions and then further up to a maximum of one hour.

How Much is Too Much?

If the highest progressions listed above sound like way too much cardio to you, you're right, they are. It is important to restate that steady cardio will only provide an extra calorie burn for a few weeks before your metabolism adjusts by slowing to compensate for it. This means the more steady cardio you add, the slower your metabolism will get. Just as reductions in calories should be minimized, so should the addition of cardio. The worst mistake you can make is cutting too many calories and adding too much cardio too quickly. Take your time to progress slowly in order to maintain your metabolism and muscle mass while you shed body fat, and always leave yourself some room to adjust when you hit plateaus at the very end of your diet. Don't be too anxious to pile on the cardio and slash calories right away to see quick results, an all too common error, as the additional hard work and deprivation will only hurt you in the long run by slowing your metabolism and by leaving you nowhere to go when progress has stopped completely.

Sample Cardio Progressions

Even at the most extreme, this plan only has a total of 3½ hours of cardio per week, and this amount should be immediately tapered back after the contest. While a very few individuals may need to do quite a bit more steady state cardio to hit their target condition, it is always important keep total, and especially steady state, cardio to a minimum when preparing for a competition. Piling on too much extra steady cardio as an easy way to cut calories will increase the amount of lean mass you lose during your diet, and slow your metabolism.

Any plan that tells you to add 2 hours of daily steady cardio right off the bat, something we've seen other trainers prescribe, should raise several red flags.

For our example client, cardio training progressed as follows.

Off-Season: Two HIIT sessions per week of 25 minutes each.

16 weeks out: Adds a third HIIT per week (biking, sprinting, or rowing).

14 weeks out: Adds one 30-minute steady cardio session before breakfast on a rest day.

11 weeks out: Fat loss had stalled, so a fourth HIIT session is added, on bike.

9 weeks out: Adds another 30-minute steady cardio session post-workout.

6 weeks out: No change in cardio (began carb cycling).

3 weeks out: For the home stretch, HIIT workouts increased to 30 minutes and steady cardio sessions increased to 45 minutes each.

Sample Strength Training Progressions

Strength training programming should change very little between the off-season and the contest preparation phase. The style of program that builds the most muscle for an athlete will also be the one which prevents the most muscle loss during a diet. If you drop the weight or the volume too much, you will send your body the message that it doesn't need to maintain that mass and it will be only too happy to let it go to conserve energy during a perceived dearth of calories.

However, your diminished ability to recover as calorie intake drops and cardio volume increases should be taken into account. Recovery is prioritized by:

- Decreasing the volume of work done at high intensity (with heavy weight)

- Decreasing the total volume
- Decreasing training frequency, if necessary

This worked for the example client as outlined below.

Off-Season to 10 weeks out: Maintains training program and continues to focus on getting new personal records for weight and repetitions on primary exercises.

9 weeks out: Reduces volume of high intensity work (greater than 80% of 1 Rep Max) from 5 to 8 sets per muscle group to 3 to 5 sets per muscle group.

6 weeks out: Decreases total training volume from 15 to 20 sets per muscle group to 10 to 15 sets.

Peak week: Specialized workout protocol.

Metabolic Maintenance

One of the major goals of the off-season is to increase your metabolic capacity so that you will more easily lose fat during your diet and avoid metabolic damage. Maintaining your metabolism while preparing for a contest should also be a top priority because:

- It will make fat loss easier and faster.
- It will allow your diet to be a lot less drastic, which will, of course, positively affect your training, mood, and personal life!
- It will prevent rapid fat gain after the contest.

Luckily, the same strategies used to increase your metabolic rate during the off-season also serve to maintain it during your diet. These are:

- Train for strength and hypertrophy. Bigger and stronger muscles = enhanced metabolic rate.

- Perform high intensity cardio, especially with long range of motion exercises like sprints, cycling, and rowing.
- Keep your calories and carbs as high as possible during your diet. Never cut 200 calories when 100 will do, and when calories start to get very low be sure to include at least one refeed day per week.
- Have a decadent 'cheat' meal once every two weeks or so during your diet. This should be just one meal (appetizer, dinner, dessert), consumed with no regrets, that gets you mentally and physically recharged rather than a several-hour binge that leaves you sick and bloated.
- Prioritize your sleep and hydration. The more depleted of fat your body becomes, the more essential these basics are to your well-being!

Posing Practice

"Posing is vitally important because, after years of hard training, working out for hours a day in the gym, and dieting with great discipline... you can win or lose a show with the same body!" - Arnold Schwarzenegger

The necessity of practicing your poses cannot be stressed enough. It's very common for competitors to put tremendous effort into their training and diet to craft a superior physique and then tack on a few posing practices in the final weeks before a show as an afterthought. This is a huge mistake! On stage, your physique is only as good as your ability to present it and the judges can only go by what they see in front of them for the 90 seconds you are on stage. They don't know how heavy you may have lifted or how tortuous your diet was; all they have to compare is a line of bodies and, where everything else is equal, presentation will win the day. We've seen many competitors backstage who were so impressive that everyone was sure they would steal the show, and been surprised time and again when they did not.

So, knowing how important posing is, how should you incorporate it into your contest prep? We are of the mind that everyone should practice his or her mandatory poses once per week, year round. This would serve to keep you sharp on your posing technique and also have the added benefit of allowing you to keep a close eye on your body fat levels year round. Once your contest prep starts, posing should be scheduled with the same consideration that you give your workouts. Seemingly effortless poses, with no apparent strain or trembling, need to be practiced...a lot. Here is a posing schedule we recommend:

Off-season: Practice posing once every one to two weeks to stay familiar with it and keep an eye on your progress. This is very conveniently done on assessment days.

16 to 20 weeks out (start of diet): Start practicing your mandatory poses three times per week for 10 to 15 minutes.

12 weeks out: Increase frequency of practice to three to five times per week and increase the duration of practice to about 20 minutes.

8 weeks out: Increase frequency of practice to five to seven times per week for 20 to 30 minutes. If your class has a routine to music, this is when you want to have it choreographed and include it in your practices.

2 weeks out through peak week: During the home stretch and especially during peak week you should pose multiple times per day. Even if the practice is not formal, hit your poses whenever and wherever you can. You want to be able to do these with your eyes closed and it also gives you an opportunity to keep a close eye on your physique during peak week.

What should your posing practice look like? This is very class-specific, so we suggest finding a video tutorial for your class on YouTube or Bodybuilding.com. Structure your posing practice around these videos and what you will be expected to do on stage. You may be holding poses for as little as 5 seconds each...or for as long as 20 seconds each, and if the competition is very close you will likely have to repeat them many times. With that in mind, practice holding your poses for 20 to 30 seconds so that on stage, for any length of time, your posing will appear effortless.

It is also essential that you hire a posing coach to evaluate you at least once during your prep as this can make a huge difference in your posing. A skilled coach will give you more beneficial feedback in one session than any amount of videos you can watch, so the more coached practices you can get in before show time the better. Use care when choosing a coach; the best coach will be either a pro or a judge in the organization you will be competing in.

Also make sure to film your posing during your weekly assessment. This will provide a much more realistic example of your presentation than pictures.

Hiring a Coach

You can, as mentioned, hire a posing coach. You also have the option of hiring a coach to oversee not only your posing but also your entire contest prep. While it's certainly possible to manage your own prep and the intent of this guide is to make it easier to do so, we would never discount the value of having a coach. Working with an expert one-on-one will provide you with a lot of benefits, some of which are:

- Personalized adjustments to all your variables to ensure you are following the best plan for your body.
- Ideally a lot of experience working with other athletes to draw on.
- Reduced stress during your prep. This can be huge - the physical stress of your diet can be tough to endure without adding to it!
- A good coach will almost always produce better results.
- Time and energy saved by having the plan done for you. This can be important if you have a busy schedule because training and cardio alone can amount to a part-time job.

There are clearly many reasons to hire a coach, and if you choose to here are some questions to ask:

- Do they have a lot of experience - success stories, etc.?
- Have they worked with athletes like you before (vegan, gluten-free, injuries, etc.)?
- Are they reasonably priced?

An excellent resource for finding coaches in your area can be found at naturalbodybuildingevents.com under 'Trainers' (http://naturalbodybuildingevents.com/trainers.html). We also offer contest preparation coaching online at veganmuscleandfitness.com under 'Online Personal Training', so if you're looking for one-on-one guidance and don't mind a distance training format utilizing Skype meetings and email, please contact us to determine availability.

Suits

Choosing a posing suit for your competition may not be at the forefront of your mind while dieting and training hard, but it can be a major source of stress if you leave it until the last minute. Depending on the organization in which you compete, your category, or your division, there may be different regulations regarding what kind of suit you should be wearing. Suits can be very expensive, so before purchasing one be sure to review the regulations of your chosen contest and, if you're still unclear, don't hesitate to contact the event coordinator for help.

For women's figure or bikini, it's an especially important aspect of your presentation. Like it or not, how well a suit flatters your skin tone and physique will factor into the judging on show day. If you're confused about which colors or cuts to choose, most custom suit designers are happy to make suggestions based on photos of yourself that you can submit via e-mail. Also keep in mind that you should order six to eight weeks in advance of your competition date, as you will definitely want the opportunity to try on your suit and send it back for alterations if necessary with plenty of time to spare. If you're on a budget, consider renting a suit or purchasing a used suit! There are several Facebook groups dedicated to selling used competition suits and accessories that you can find by searching the words "competition suits". For a custom suit, you will need to take careful measurements to submit to the designer, who will also take into consideration your target stage weight when creating the suit. If you are purchasing or renting a used suit or purchasing a new suit that is not custom fitted, you will need to size it according to your target stage weight.

There are many options available that can be found via internet search. Here are a few that our friends or we have used, covering a wide range of budgets:

Bodybuilding.com

cherrybombs.net

competitionsuits.com

suitsbyamy.com

lidiaconti.com

cariesposingsuits.com

Tanning

Your contest tan is so much more important than you'd think! It's common for new competitors to get a regular spray tan or, worse, no tan at all for their first contest and learn the hard way that stage lights are so bright that they can make even the darkest natural tan look ghostly pale, washing out all muscle definition. Your skin needs to be as dark as you can get it! At the Naturally Fit Super Show in Austin, in which we both competed in 2013, we were actually scored on our tans according to the critiques we received after the show. Two options available to you are purchasing spray tanning that is coordinated by the show organizers, or using a self-tanner.

Many shows now offer onsite tanning for athletes, which is convenient and likely to be as dark as you need. The problem with getting a spray tan outside of a competition lies in getting across just how dark you need to be, which is far darker than they ordinarily tan people! At the venue, it'll be understood, although you can always ask for another coat. If you choose this route, be sure to schedule it well in advance so you can get a desirable time slot. Also plan to thoroughly exfoliate your skin every other day of the week prior. This will help the tan adhere to your skin and prevent streaks and blotches that can mar your presentation. Also, if backstage touch-ups are available, get them done an hour before hitting the stage.

Self-tanners are also available that will get you as dark as you need and save you some serious cash. A great brand with vegan ingredients is Pro Tan, and it's available at Bodybuilding.com. The downsides of this approach include the fact that you will need to begin applying it daily at least five days before the show, which means a lot of work and inconvenience for both you and likely a friend who will get the hard to reach places. You'll also be going about your daily business looking bizarre throughout the week. However, it is cheap, effective if properly done, and will save you the stress of fitting in an hour or more of standing around with other competitors and tanning employees in the nude during the final hours of contest prep.

On the last note, men may want to make sure to bring an old posing suit or a thong to wear for spray tanning in case there are no paper suits provided. Derek has experienced everything from being the only nude man facing a line of clothed competitors waiting to be tanned (thereafter being referred to as "that naked guy" backstage), to wearing an infant's sock, so he stresses that coming prepared to your tanning session is important!

Posing Oil

Just like a good contest tan, the right posing oil can transform your physique by enhancing its definition and muscularity. The wrong oil can be even worse than none at all, though, so some caution is warranted before you apply!

Glazes are often included with a contest tanning package, and you can be sure these will have the right level of sheen as well as some expectation that it will be properly applied by professionals. This is a great option because you don't need to worry about doing anything more than showing up 20 to 30 minutes before going onstage so that it can be applied.

If you are using a self-tanner, then tanning products such as Muscle Juice by Pro Tan are available online, but they can be expensive and will need to be applied by a friend at the show. Shea butter or baby oil can also work; but be sure to blot off any areas that go on too thickly. A helper to make sure that it's even and to apply it on your back is a must! A popular option has always been cooking spray such as Pam, but we don't advise it. Some venues have actually banned its use due to slipperiness on floors and it tends to be too thick and shiny, giving you a strange, saran-wrapped appearance.

Show Day Packing List

Since you will be coated in faux tan and oil during your show it's a good idea to bring along some clothes, towels, and sheets if you're staying in a hotel so that you don't spread stains all over the venue and hotel room. Pack:

- one or two cover-up outfits including sandals, dark-colored loose pants, and a dark-colored loose long-sleeved shirt with no zippers
- black sheets for the bed
- one or more towels for blotting oil after the contest
- exfoliating body wash and a wash cloth or scrub brush both for preparing for your tan and removing your tan after the show
- your music for the routine, if necessary
- all the food and water you need for your planned meals

Receiving Feedback

Once the show is over, make sure you stick around to get feedback from the judges as discussed in the next section! This will help you plan for your next competition.

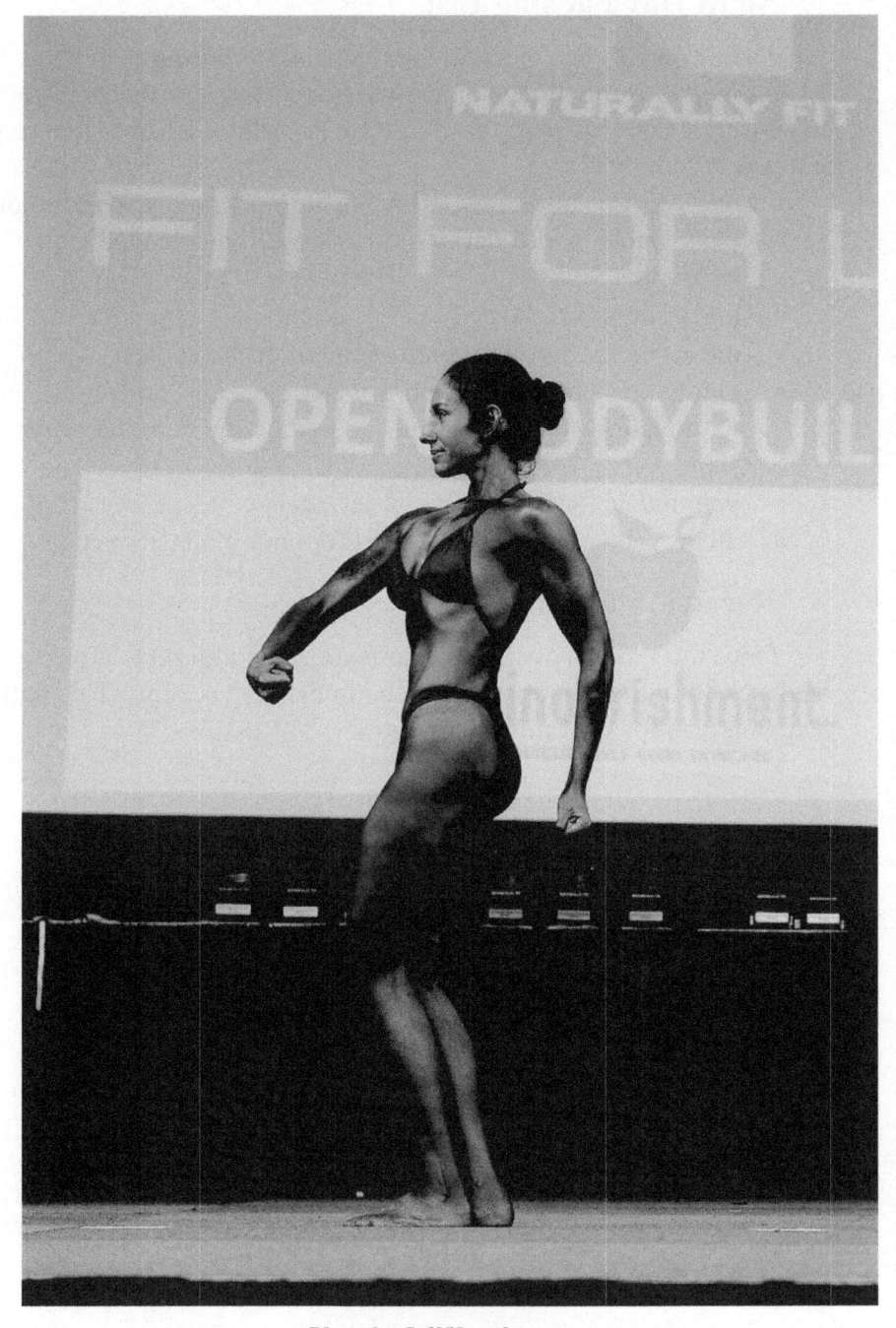

Photo by Jeff Kutscher

Section 3: Peak Week

There are many strategies out there to help a physique athlete look his or her best on show day and untangling them all to choose the best (and healthiest) methods will take some legwork. Investigate your options ahead of time and choose wisely rather than allowing last minute panic to dictate your choices. We have tried several approaches and very much prefer the moderate peaking techniques popularized by Dr. Layne Norton. Many of the recommendations in this section are based on our experiences with his recommendations for contest peak week and, while there are many other popular approaches, it is our opinion that these methods carry the least risk for the greatest benefit.

It is important to note that you should already be in show condition by the beginning of peak week. That's why the assessments of the preceding weeks are so important; making adjustments as needed prevents panic-driven decisions to make drastic changes at the last minute, and spares you unnecessary stress. These peak week strategies are designed to help your body look rested, recovered, and vital after a hard diet - not to burn another few ounces of body fat off.

Chapter 10: Peak Week Nutrition

Just as you've done for the rest of the year, during peak week you will focus on manipulating the amounts of protein, carbohydrates, and fat that you are taking in to help your body look its best.

Two primary objectives of peak week are to 'fill out' your muscles as much as possible without making them look 'soft' or 'spilled over'. This is done to avoid looking 'flat' or 'stringy'. What does all this mean?! Much of a muscle's volume (how big it looks) can be attributed to stored carbohydrates in the form of glycogen, and water. After many weeks of eating a calorie deficit and doing extra cardio to shed fat, muscle glycogen levels are very low which also reduces muscle water levels and can leave your physique looking thin and deflated. During peak week, diet and exercise parameters are adjusted to help reverse this process and make your physique look lean, muscular, and vital.

Muscular Dictionary

Full/Filled-Out: When your muscles are full of stored glycogen and water they look much bigger and harder. You'll notice the difference after a cheat meal.

Soft/Spilled-Over: More is not necessarily better as far as carbohydrates are concerned, and consuming them past an optimal point can make a physique look less defined, or soft and puffy.

Flat/Stringy: This describes a depleted body with low muscle glycogen and intracellular water levels, which looks deflated and wiry. It can usually be quickly improved by drinking water and consuming sodium and carbohydrate rich foods.

Peak Week Macronutrients

By the time you reach your final week your diet is likely very restricted, with low calories and probably low carbohydrates and fats as well. Many peaking methods involve further reducing your diet for the first half of the week then massively increasing your carbohydrate intake in the final days (or hours) before the contest in the hopes of a dramatic rebound, with your body 'super-compensating' its carbohydrate stores after having been so depleted. This may seem like sound logic but it is quite risky and will just as often result in a flat and stringy appearance or a soft and puffy one as it will a filled-out physique, and the risk is totally unnecessary. Instead of complex and risky nutritional manipulation, we prefer to slowly and gradually increase carbohydrates over the entire final week, giving your body plenty of time to adjust to the diet change and come in full and replenished. Instead of risking it all to look perhaps 2% better, why not guarantee that you'll get on stage at 98%?

It's also important to note that there are no ideal recommendations that will suit everyone; your own optimal protocol can only develop through several attempts, trial and error, and taking lots of notes.

How to Adjust Your Diet

While it is still very important to increase carbohydrates and restore muscle glycogen, it is much more practical to start increasing at the very start of the final week rather than at the eleventh hour. Assuming your show is on a Saturday, here are our recommended dietary adjustments, based on Layne Norton's front-loading principles for peaking.

Saturday and Sunday, One Week Out:

Protein: Decrease your dieting amount by about 5-10%

Carbs: Increase from your dieting amount by about 30%

Fat: Maintain at dieting level (low)

Monday, Five Days Out:

Protein: Decrease by another 5-10%

Carbs: Increase by another 50-75% (this is your largest refeed day)

Fat: Increase by 5-10%

Tuesday, Four Days Out:

Protein: Increase by 5%

Carbs: Decrease by about 20% (you are now at about 2 times your diet level)

Fat: Same as Monday

Wednesday, Three Days Out:

Protein: Increase by 5% (back to Saturday/Sunday level)

Carbs: Decrease by another 20% (you are now at about 1.5 times your diet level)

Fat: Decrease by 5-10% (back to diet level)

Thursday, Two Days Out:

Protein: Increase by 5% (around the same as diet level)

Carbs: Decrease by another 20% (back to Saturday/Sunday level)

Fat: Same as Wednesday

Friday, One Day Out:

Amounts here can vary widely. By starting the week very high and then slowly tapering back your body should have plenty of time to recover and fill out. So use Friday as an extra day to: increase intakes if you're still looking flat, hold steady if you're looking good, or cut back a little if you're looking bloated or puffy.

For example, if you're looking great or need to fill out slightly:

Protein: Increase by 5%

Carbs: Increase by 25%

Fats: Maintain

You can use the previous days in the week as a guide in modifying your diet to your current needs. If you have more filling out to do, duplicate Monday or Tuesday on Friday. If you're looking too full, take Friday at your diet levels and finally, if you look perfect then duplicate Thursday's numbers.

Saturday, Show Day:

The goal on Saturday is to take it easy and eliminate any potential risky variables, ensuring that you look rested, confident, and ready. It's a good idea to get up early on Saturday so you have more time to get in several meals and some light activity so that you are fully alert for prejudging. Use Thursday's macronutrient breakdown and try to eat your first meal of the day 6 to 8 hours before you'll be onstage. This usually means having breakfast around 6 A.M. As with all your days, divide the nutrients of the day as evenly as possible over five to six meals, eating every two to three hours. Here are some guidelines:

- Your third or fourth meal of the day (roughly two hours before stepping on the stage) should be a 'fill-out' meal unless you're already very filled out. Have a larger and more refined meal here with about double the carbs and fat of your other meals as well as a liberal amount of sodium. A meal Derek has had in the past that meets these guidelines was a large submarine sandwich with vegan mayonnaise, Tofurkey (faux meat) slices, and vegetables on white bread, but you should tailor it to your needs and preference. Think of this meal as topping off your glycogen tanks.

- The closer you get to stage time, the simpler and more easily digested your meals should be to avoid indigestion or bloating. Most competitors, for example, eat rice cakes with peanut butter and jelly.
- If you still need to fill out, eat a quick carbs and fat meal such as a vegan candy bar about 10 to 15 minutes before going on stage. Eating some concentrated sodium may also help. We tend to be very skeptical of last minute tricks, but something this minor is unlikely to cause harm and might help.
- Be careful to limit or avoid any foods that can cause bloating such as legumes and cruciferous vegetables. Stick to easily digested foods such as rice, sweet potatoes, fruit and tofu.

Chapter 11: Peak Week Training

You may have noticed a theme in our peak week recommendations: that deviating too much from your established routine immediately before your contest is generally not desirable, and the same holds true here. We recommend sticking with your existing training plan right up until a few days before the show. This will keep you feeling strong and full, aid in recovery, help deliver nutrients from your peak week diet to your muscles, and prevent you from getting too stressed from a change in routine. The only changes should be to decrease the weights you ordinarily use to prevent being overly sore or getting injured, and to switch to a total body circuit at the end of the week in order to aid recovery and nutrient delivery to your muscles.

Another consideration is to make sure your final leg day occurs 10 to 14 days before the show. This is because leg day is the most strenuous workout in anyone's rotation, so it causes the most systemic inflammation and require the most time to recover. Any inflammation on the day of the show can leave you looking soft and puffy rather than crisply defined and legs that aren't fully recovered may not look as big and muscular. You also don't want to be flexing sore legs on stage, so give your legs a long rest before show day. Don't worry, the light peak week exercise and extra calories will keep you from losing any muscle! Here is an example of a peak week training schedule:

Friday, Saturday, and Sunday, About One Week Out:

Continue with existing program, but decrease loads by about 75% of normal and take no sets to failure. Continue with diet levels of cardio.

Monday, Five Days Out:

Continue to train as above. Reduce cardio to 75% of dieting levels, with no more HIIT from here on out.

Tuesday, Four Days Out:

Continue to train as above. Reduce cardio to 50% of dieting levels.

Wednesday. Three Days Out:

Continue to train as above. Reduce cardio to 25% of dieting level.

Thursday and Friday, Two and Three Days Out:

Do 30 to 45 minutes of circuit training using one exercise per muscle group and performing 10 to 20 reps per set at about 60% of your usual weights. This is just to keep delivering glycogen to the muscles and aid in recovery, not to break personal lifting records, so it should not be too strenuous! Only 10 to 20 minutes of steady cardio is necessary today.

Saturday, Show Day:

Perform a pumping up workout after Meal 1, after your 'fill-out' meal, and about 10 minutes before going onstage. How to pump up is outlined in the following section. The only cardio you should perform today is walking or light jogging around the venue to settle your nerves!

Pump Workout

A pump workout is a light circuit program designed to fill your muscles with blood right before going on stage. It can also be done earlier on show day to help bring nutrients to your muscles. It strategically targets muscles that are the easiest (and most impressive) to get a pump in such as chest, delts, and arms. You're not reaching for a huge pump like one you'd strive for in the gym, as it would wash out all of your definition; your objective here is enhancement, so a brief 5 to 10 minute light circuit is all you want to do. We've seen competitors pump up intensely for 30 minutes before going onstage and this seemed like a great way to get over-pumped and exhausted before it's even time to pose. Err on the side of too little and spare yourself energy for the real work at hand!

Every venue provides different equipment to the competitors so it is difficult to plan based on what might be available. It's a good idea to plan on doing bodyweight exercises and to bring a set of resistance bands for rows, laterals, and curls in case no equipment is provided or available. Some general guidelines for a pump routine are:

- Keep it 5 to 10 minutes long.
- Focus on chest, delts, and arms as those are the easiest to pump up and a pump will be most noticeable for these muscles.
- Do not pump up your legs. Any leg pump will obscure definition that you worked too hard for.
- Be mindful of your tan! Don't lie down or perform any movements that cause your skin to rub or chafe.
- For weighted exercises, use a light to moderate weight for 10 to 30 reps and keep rest intervals to around 30 seconds.
- Try to work abs into your pumping circuit. Most people neglect abs here, but getting a couple of sets in can really make your midsection definition pop a bit more and have a big impact.

Here's an example of a pump workout using bodyweight, bands, and dumbbells:

Push-ups
Dumbbell Lateral Raise
Band Rows

Dumbbell Bicep Curl
One-Arm Dumbbell Extension
Bench Tuck (abs)

Perform exercises in a circuit, for 10 to 30 reps per exercise (well short of failure), with rests of 30 seconds between exercises and between circuits - unless you are getting fatigued, then rest longer. Keep constant tension on the muscles with no rest at bottom or top of reps and really squeeze. Two to three circuits should be sufficient.

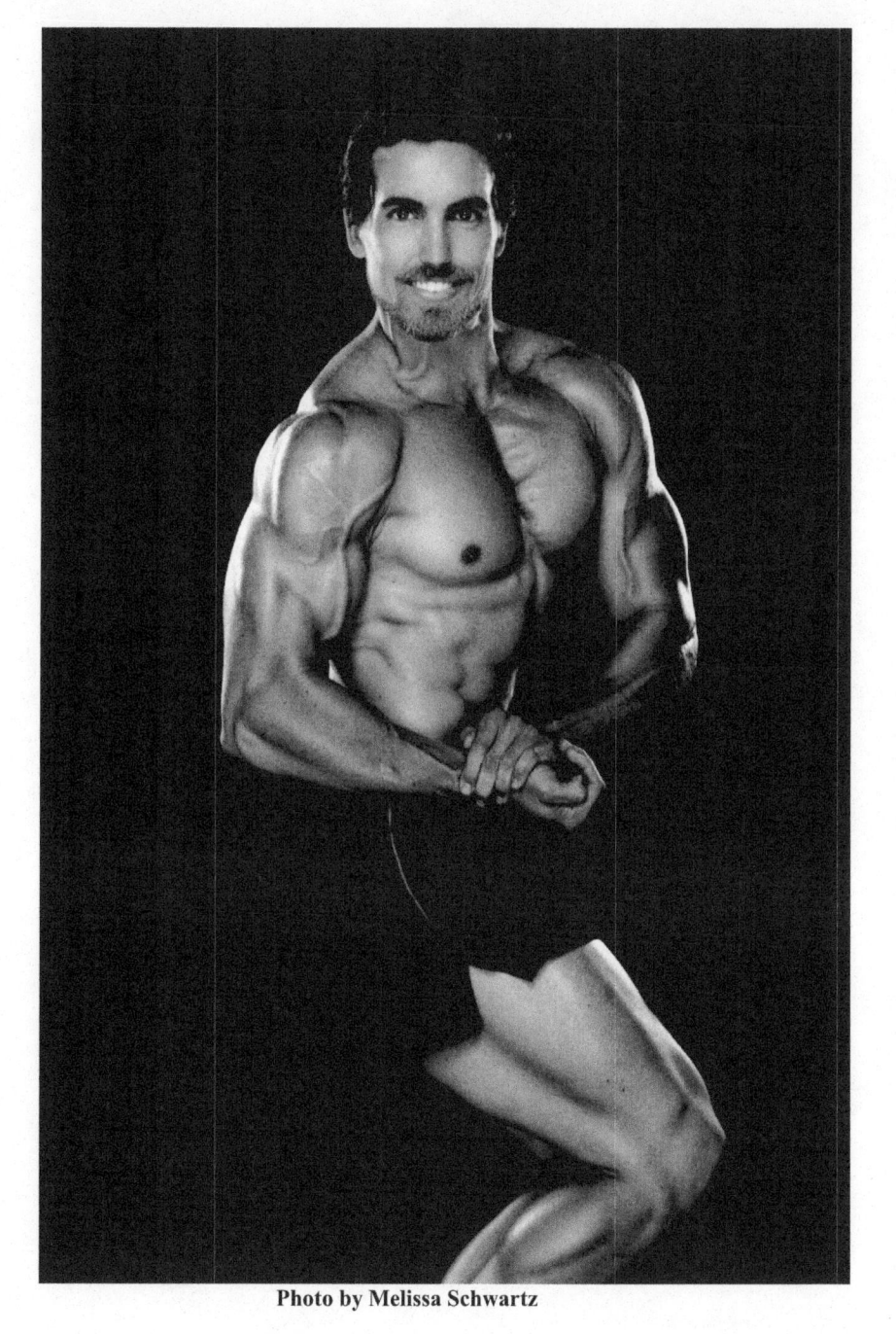

Photo by Melissa Schwartz

Section 4: Post-Contest

If you're reading this after your competition - congratulations! Stepping on a stage as a physique athlete takes a phenomenal amount of work, dedication, and courage. As a vegan, you also had an important message to send, which adds a whole other level of effort! You've spent the last four to six months preparing your body for this event and, hopefully, you placed as well as your efforts merited. So now what?

The post-contest phase of bodybuilding receives little attention but it is an extremely important part of the cycle: time to reflect on your performance, set future goals, and give yourself the best possible start to a successful off-season. There are a lot of physiological, psychological, and social pressures working against you at this time, so it's important to have a plan in place.

Chapter 12: After the Show

Reverse Dieting

If you're coming off a long and restrictive diet, all of the foods you've been craving for months will be the first thing on your mind and the friends and family who have been waiting for you to be able to indulge with them will be all too willing to facilitate a post-contest binge. In fact, it's a tradition for competitors to binge on junk food for days or even weeks following a contest but, as you might expect, this can seriously derail your off-season. As discussed previously, the systematic reductions in calories and increases in steady cardio training have slowly lowered your metabolic rate. Your body makes this adjustment naturally to prevent starvation, and the consequence is that now your basal metabolic rate is likely about half of what it was before your diet. Halting all exercise and going on an eating spree in this condition is a great way to rapidly gain fat, leaving you at a higher percentage body fat with a slower metabolic rate and suboptimal hormone profile, none of which spells a good start to the off-season. Yes, a treat meal can stimulate your metabolism and is a useful diet tool but it only takes an extra meal or two for your calorie intake to surpass any metabolic bump. So what's a starving, post-contest bodybuilder to do?

Our suggestion is to allow yourself one to three treat meals over the next three to four days, making sure that all other meals are small, light, and nutrient dense just as they were during your diet. This will allow you to sate your cravings and spend some time celebrating your achievement without too much backsliding. After this three to four day period, your best chance for long-term success will come from a properly planned reverse diet.

A reverse diet is the exact opposite of a pre-contest diet. It's focus is on slowly increasing calories in the weeks and months after a contest with the objective of recovering (or even improving) your off-season metabolic rate, keeping body fat gain to a minimum, and improving your chances of an overall productive off-season. These guidelines, which we first saw published by Dr. Layne Norton, bodybuilder and PhD in Nutritional Science, have worked for us and for our clients and cover each aspect of the goals listed above.

Using your nutrient values from the week prior to peak week as a reference, reduce your daily protein intake by about 10 percent, increase your carbohydrate intake by about 40 percent, and your fat intake by about 10 percent. After your initial treat meals, eat no more of them for at least three to four weeks. Reduce cardio to two times per week, preferably of HIIT. You should also return to your regular lifting schedule after taking three days to one week off and.

In the first week you should expect a small amount of weight gain, but by the second week you should see a slight drop in weight as your metabolic rate responds. Once you see this weight drop, add around 20 grams of daily carbohydrates and maintain this level until you notice another small drop in weight. This usually takes about one to three weeks.

Over the next 10 weeks increase carbs by 5 to 25 daily grams per week and fat by up to five grams per week depending on how your metabolism is responding. Make small increases if you're gaining or maintaining weight and large ones if you continue to see drops in weight.

After this 12-week reverse diet, consider yourself in full off-season mode and follow the nutrition recommendations from that section.

Setting Future Goals

As we now know, setting specific, objective goals and regularly assessing your progress is essential for success in this sport. Now that you've completed a contest you have an essential new tool in your arsenal: experience. This will greatly aid you in future planning as you reflect on your experiences of each phase of the process to decide what could be improved. Here are some questions you can ask yourself that will help you shape your goals for your next contest:

- *What did the judges label as your strengths and weaknesses?* In most competitions, the judges will provide you with a scorecard or verbal feedback, and it is definitely in your best interest to take advantage of this!
- *How was your posing?* Posing is so incredibly important, and is always a great aspect of your training to target for extra work because everyone can improve here. Take some time to go through contest photos or videos, or your latest assessment photos and videos, and analyze your best and worst poses...then commit to making them your best.
- *How was your conditioning?* Did you take the stage full, shredded, and vascular or were you still looking soft in places? Maybe you were very lean, but you looked flat and stringy. Make careful, objective notes.
- *How was your overall shape and symmetry?* Seeing pictures of yourself next to other competitors is one of the best ways to determine your proportions and your strengths and weaknesses. Were your shoulders too narrow? Were your thighs too small? For example, after Derek's first contest the judges gave him feedback that he needed more muscle size overall, but especially in his arms and legs. He factored that into his program design, and within a year he was able to improve them enough to place first. Find your weak points, and then plan your off-season around improving them.
- *Were you big enough?* This question applies mostly to male and female bodybuilders. How was your level of muscularity compared to the competition? Do you just need to maintain your current level of muscularity and improve your posing and conditioning or could you honestly stand to gain 10 to 15 pounds of muscle to be more competitive? Take notes and plan accordingly.

Now is also an excellent time to review your notes from your off-season, pre-contest, and peak week phases. Go over them while your contest is fresh in your mind and make notes on what worked well and what needs to change. Once you have addressed these questions, you should be forming some very clear goals for each phase of your next competition. Write them down and, where applicable, break them down into incremental two to four week goals (for example, add ¼ inch to thighs or gain two lean pounds). Regularly assess your progress to stay on track and change direction with your diet and training as needed.

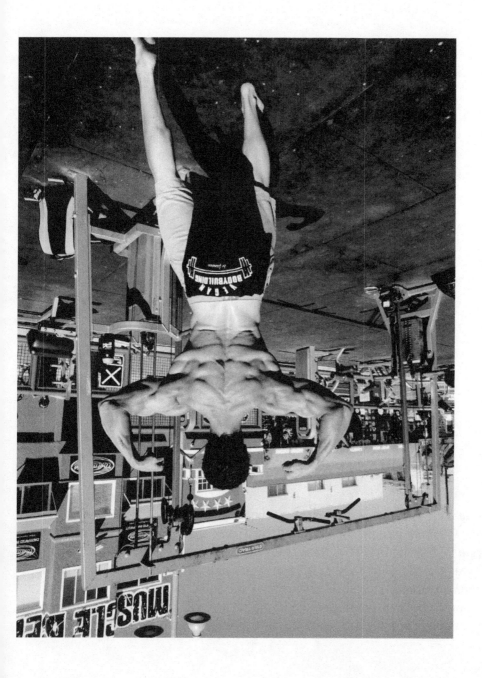

Appendix 1: Our 2013 Journals

Derek Tresize

Goals: Derek's goal was to stay lean while gaining as much muscle as possible. He also trained around several injuries. At the completion of this program, he met his goal, winning first place in the Men's Bodybuilding division in the Light-Heavyweight class.

Training Philosophy: Frequency during the off-season was 4 to 5 training days per week, with a 3-day split routine. Rep ranges were varied each workout to work both slow and fast twitch muscle fiber types by alternating rep schemes A and B week to week.

During the pre-contest phase, frequency was increased to 5 training days every week. When calories started getting challengingly low, approximately one less set per exercise was performed to reduce volume and improve recovery.

Derek often substitutes exercises (for example, front squat instead of squat or barbell row instead of dumbbell row), but the same basic movements are always performed. Consistency and intensity are more important than exercise variety.

Also, variations to increase intensity and keep the routines interesting were often performed, such as supersets, German volume sets, or rest pause sets. These were generally limited to one or two exercises in a given workout, for about half of overall workouts.

Derek's Training Program

Day 1: Chest, Back, and Abs

Exercise	Sets	Reps A	Reps B
Weighted Pull-ups	5	8	12
Dumbbell Row	4	10	15

Exercise			
Deadlift	4	10	20
Bench Press	5	5	8-12
Dumbbell Incline Press	4	6-8	12
Decline Pullovers	3	10	12
Plank Position	3	Failure	Failure

Day 2: Shoulders and Arms

Exercise	Sets	Reps A	Reps B
Bent-over Dumbbell Laterals	4	8	15
Military Press	5	5	12
Seated Dumbbell Laterals	4	8	15
Preacher Curl	5	8	15
Dumbbell Incline Curl	4	10	15
Skullcrushers	5	8	15
Cable Pushdown	4	10	15

Day 3: Legs and Abs

Exercise	Sets	Reps A	Reps B
Standing Calf Raise	5	8	20
Squat	5	8-12	15-20
Lunges	4	10	15
Leg Extension	4	10	25
Romanian Deadlift	4	10	15
Leg Curl	4	10	20
Bicycle Crunches	3	30	30

Derek's Off-Season Meal Plan

Weight: 198 lbs
Body Fat: 10%

Meals and subsequent values varied day-to-day, and approximately two meals out were eaten per week.

Breakfast:
¾ Cup Steel Cut Oats
1 Banana

Calories: 571
Protein: 16
Carbs: 112
Fat: 8

Pre-Workout:
1 Serving Vega Pre-Workout Energizer

Post-Workout:
1 Banana
1 Scoop PlantFusion Protein
1 Cup Soymilk

Calories: 301
Protein: 28
Carbs: 41
Fat: 4

Mid-Morning:
1 Banana
1 Cup Soymilk
½ Scoop Vega One Protein
¾ Cup Cannellini Beans
⅛ Cup Flax Seeds
½ Cup Oatmeal
1 Cup Spinach
½ Cup Strawberries

Calories: 678
Protein: 37
Carbs: 105

Fat: 15

Lunch:
½ Head Romaine
Additional Raw Vegetable Salad Toppings (Cucumber, Tomato, Etc.)
Balsamic Vinegar

1 Sweet Potato
2 Bowls (About Cups) Red Lentil Soup
⅛ Bunch Broccoli, cooked
¼ Block Extra Firm Tofu

Calories: 674
Protein: 43
Carbs: 111
Fat: 8

Afternoon:
1 Banana
1 Cup Soymilk
½ Scoop Vega One Protein
¾ Cup Cannellini Beans
⅛ Cup Flax Seeds
½ Cup Oatmeal
1 Cup Spinach
½ Cup Strawberries

Calories: 678
Protein: 37
Carbs: 105
Fat: 15

Dinner:
1 Head Romaine

¼ Block Extra Firm Tofu
⅓ Cup Uncooked Brown Rice

½ Can Black Beans, Rinsed
¼ Bunch Broccoli, Cooked
½ Avocado

Calories: 793
Protein: 37
Carbs: 112
Fat: 20

Totals:

Calories: 3791
Protein: 197 g
Carbs: 612 g
Fat: 68 g

20% Protein
65% Carbohydrates
15% Fat

Derek's Early Pre-Contest Meal Plan

Weight: 193 lbs
Body Fat: 7%

Meals and subsequent values varied day-to-day, and approximately one meal out was eaten per week.

Breakfast:
1 Cup Oatmeal
¼ Cup Blueberries

Calories: 321
Protein: 10
Carbs: 59
Fat: 6

Pre-Workout:
    1 Serving Vega Pre-Workout Energizer
    ½ Serving Kre-Alkalyn Creatine

Post-Workout:
    1 Banana
    1 Scoop PlantFusion Protein
    1 Cup Soymilk
    ½ Serving Kre-Alkalyn Creatine

    Calories: 301
    Protein: 28
    Carbs: 41
    Fat: 4

Mid-Morning:
    ½ Banana
    1 Cup Soymilk
    1/2 Plant Fusion Protein
    1 Cup Cannellini Beans
    ⅛ Pumpkin Seeds
    1 Cup Spinach
    ½ Cup Strawberries

    Calories: 532
    Protein: 40
    Carbs: 76
    Fat: 10

Lunch:
    ½ Head Romaine
    Additional Raw Vegetable Salad Toppings (Cucumber, Tomato, Etc.)
    Balsamic Vinegar

    1 Sweet Potato
    2 Bowls (About 3 Cups) Red Lentil Soup
    ⅛ Bunch Broccoli, Cooked

½ Block Extra Firm Tofu

Calories: 771
Protein: 53
Carbs: 114
Fat: 13

Afternoon:
½ Banana
1 Cup Soymilk
1/2 Plant Fusion Protein
1 Cup Cannellini Beans
⅛ Pumpkin Seeds
1 Cup Spinach
½ Cup Strawberries

Calories: 532
Protein: 40
Carbs: 76
Fat: 10

Dinner:
1 Head Romaine

½ Block Extra Firm Tofu
1/6 Cup Uncooked Brown Rice
½ Can Black Beans, Rinsed
½ Bunch Broccoli, Cooked

Calories: 595
Protein: 42
Carbs: 82
Fat: 11

Totals:

Calories: 2959
Protein: 208 g
Carbs: 444 g

Fat: 46 g

25% Protein
60% Carbohydrates
15% Fat

Derek's Late Pre-Contest Meal Plan

Weight: 187 lbs
Body Fat: 4%

Meals and subsequent values varied day-to-day. Refeed days with extra carbohydrates and reduced fat and protein were eaten one day per week. Every other week this day included a decadent meal out.

Breakfast:
1 Cup Oat Bran

Calories: 480
Protein: 21
Carbs: 72
Fat: 11

Pre-Workout:
1 Serving Vega Pre-Workout Energizer
½ Serving Kre-Alkalyn Creatine
1 Serving BCAAs

Post-Workout:
1 Kiwi
1 Scoop PlantFusion Protein
1 Cup Unsweetened Soymilk
½ Serving Kre-Alkalyn Creatine

Calories: 236
Protein: 29
Carbs: 18
Fat: 6

Mid-Morning:
1 Cup Unsweetened Soymilk
¾ Scoop Plant Fusion Protein
1 Cup Cannellini Beans
1 Cup Spinach
¼ Cup Oat Bran

Calories: 500
Protein: 46
Carbs: 63
Fat: 8

Lunch:
½ Head Romaine
Additional Raw Vegetable Salad Toppings (Cucumber, Tomato, Etc.)
Balsamic Vinegar

1 ½ Bowls (About 2 ¼ Cups) Red Lentil Soup
⅛ Bunch Broccoli, cooked

Calories: 344
Protein: 24
Carbs: 58
Fat: 2

Afternoon:
1 Cup Unsweetened Soymilk
¾ Scoop Plant Fusion Protein
1 Cup Cannellini Beans
1 Cup Spinach
¼ Cup Oat Bran

Calories: 500
Protein: 46
Carbs: 63
Fat: 8

Dinner:

1 Head Romaine

½ Block Extra Firm Tofu
¼ Bunch Broccoli, Cooked
3 Ounces Seitan

Calories: 364
Protein: 47
Carbs: 21
Fat: 11

Totals:

Calories: 2424
Protein: 213 g
Carbs: 295 g
Fat: 45 g

35% Protein
50% Carbohydrates
15% Fat

Marcella Torres

Goals: Marcella was eight months post-pregnancy when she began her contest prep. Fat loss was our priority when designing her program, as she was about 29% fat and needed to hit an aggressive target of at least 12% to be competitive in the bodybuilding category. While there wasn't sufficient time to regain much of the muscle lost during pregnancy, she met her fat loss goal and placed second in the Women's Bodybuilding division in the Lightweight class.

Training Philosophy: Frequency during the off-season and pre-contest was 5 training days per week, alternating between two 3-day split routines for added exercise and workout structure variety. Rep ranges were varied each workout to work both slow and fast twitch muscle fiber types by alternating rep schemes A and B week to week.

During the pre-contest period, frequency was kept at 5 training days every week. When calories started getting challengingly low, approximately one less set per exercise was performed to reduce volume and improve recovery, and lower rep ranges were emphasized to maintain strength and muscle mass.

Marcella followed two alternating routines to have more exercise variety built into her program, but all variations were based upon the same basic movements. Consistency and intensity are more important than exercise variety.

Also, variations to increase intensity and keep the routines interesting were often performed, such as supersets, German volume sets, or rest pause sets. Supersets were used to increase calorie expenditure during her weight-lifting sessions and are indicated with an indent: the indented exercise is superset with the exercise above.

Marcella's Training Program

Day 1: Chest, Back, and Abs

Exercise	Sets	Reps A	Reps B
Assisted Pull-ups	5	8	12
Barbell Row	4	8	15
Straight Arm Pulldown	4	10	15
Bench Press	5	5	8-12
Dumbbell Incline Press	4	6-8	15
Dumbbell Fly	4	8	15
Heel drags	4	20	20
V-Ups	4	15	15

Day 2: Shoulders and Triceps

Exercise	Sets	Reps A	Reps B
Bodyweight Reverse Fly	4	8	15
Military Press	4	10	15
Arnold Press	3	8	12
Seated Dumbbell Laterals	3	8	15
Reverse Grip Bench Press	4	8	12
Cable Pushdown	4	8	15
Dumbbell Overhead Extension	3	8	15

Day 3: Legs and Biceps

Exercise	Sets	Reps A	Reps B
Lunges	4	10	15
Squat	4	8	12
Leg Curl	4	8	20
Romanian Deadlift	4	8	12
Seated Calf Press	6	12	20
Alternating Dumbbell Curl	4	5	12
Barbell Curl	5	8	15

Day 4: Chest, Shoulders, and Abs

Exercise	Sets	Reps A	Reps B
Incline Bench Press	4	8	12
Dumbbell Bench Press	3	8	15
Cable Cross	4	10	15
Lying Rear/Side	3	10	15

Laterals			
Barbell Front Raise	3	8	12
Dumbbell Shoulder Press	4	10	15
Bicycle Crunches	3	30	30
Plank	3	Failure	Failure

Day 5: Back and Arms

Exercise	Sets	Reps A	Reps B
Pulldowns	3	8	15
Close Grip Bench	3	8	15
T-Bar Row	4	10	15
Bench Dips	4	8	15
Dumbbell Row	4	8	15
Preacher Curl	4	10	20
Incline Curl	3	10	15
Cable Pushdown	3	8	15

Day 6: Legs and Abs

Exercise	Sets	Reps A	Reps B
Squat	4	12	20
Leg Press	4	10	15
Leg Extension	4	10	20
Romanian Deadlift	3	8	20
Single-Leg Calf Raise	4	10	20
Calf Press	4	15	30
V-Ups	3	20	20
Crunches	3	30	30

Marcella's Off-Season Meal Plan

Weight: 140 lbs
Body Fat: 29%

Meals and subsequent values varied day-to-day, and approximately two meals out were eaten per week.

Breakfast:
>1 Cup Light Soymilk
>½ Scoop PlantFusion Protein
>½ Banana
>½ Cup Strawberries
>
>½ Cup Oat Bran
>¼ Cup Blueberries
>
>Calories: 480
>Protein: 28
>Carbs: 75
>Fat: 8

Post-Workout:
>½ Scoop PlantFusion Protein
>1 Cup Soymilk
>
>Calories: 120
>Protein: 17
>Carbs: 8
>Fat: 3

Mid-Morning:
>½ Banana
>½ Cup Soymilk
>¼ Cup Cannellini Beans

1/16 Cup Raw Hulled Pumpkin Seeds
¼ Cup Strawberries

Calories: 226
Protein: 11
Carbs: 36
Fat: 6

Lunch:
½ Head Romaine
¼ Block Extra Firm Tofu
Additional Raw Vegetable Salad Toppings (Cucumber, Tomato, Etc.)
Balsamic Vinegar

1 Sweet Potato
1 Bowl (About 1½ Cups) Red Lentil Soup
⅛ Bunch Broccoli, cooked

Calories: 484
Protein: 31
Carbs: 82
Fat: 7

Afternoon:
½ Banana
½ Cup Soymilk
¼ Cup Cannellini Beans
1/16 Cup Raw Hulled Pumpkin Seeds
¼ Cup Strawberries

Calories: 226
Protein: 11
Carbs: 36
Fat: 6

Dinner:
½ Head Romaine (Salad)

½ Block Extra Firm Tofu
¼ Cup Uncooked Brown Rice
¼ Cup Edamame
¼ Bunch Broccoli, Cooked

Calories: 497
Protein: 36
Carbs: 54
Fat: 14

Totals:

Calories: 2365
Protein: 155 g
Carbs: 335 g
Fat: 48 g

25% Protein
60% Carbohydrates
15% Fat

Marcella's Early Pre-Contest Meal Plan

Weight: 132 lbs
Body Fat: 24%

Meals and subsequent values varied day-to-day, and approximately one meal out was eaten per week.

Breakfast:

1/3 Cup Oat Bran
1/8 Cup Blueberries
¼ Block Extra Firm Tofu

Calories: 265
Protein: 17

Carbs: 29
Fat: 8

Post-Workout:
> 1 Scoop PlantFusion Protein

> Calories: 301
> Protein: 28
>> Carbs: 41
>> Fat: 4

Mid-Morning:
> ½ Banana
> ½ Cup Soymilk
> ½ Scoop Plant Fusion Protein
> ½ Cup Cannellini Beans
> ⅛ Pumpkin Seeds

> Calories: 270
> Protein: 27
> Carbs: 29
> Fat: 4

Lunch:
> ½ Head Romaine
> Additional Raw Vegetable Salad Toppings (Cucumber, Tomato, Etc.)
> ¼ Block Extra Firm Tofu
> Balsamic Vinegar

> ½ Sweet Potato
> 1½ Bowl (About 2¼ Cups) Red Lentil Soup
> ⅛ Bunch Broccoli, cooked

> Calories: 478
> Protein: 35
> Carbs: 78
> Fat: 7

Afternoon:
  ½ Banana
  ½ Cup Soymilk
  ½ Scoop Plant Fusion Protein
  ½ Cup Cannellini Beans
  ⅛ Pumpkin Seeds

  Calories: 270
  Protein: 27
  Carbs: 29
  Fat: 4

Dinner:
  ½ Head Romaine (Salad)

  ½ Block Extra Firm Tofu
  1/8 Cup Uncooked Brown Rice
  1/3 Cup Edamame
  ¼ Bunch Broccoli, Cooked

  Calories: 465
  Protein: 37
  Carbs: 44
  Fat: 18

Totals:

  Calories: 1868
  Protein: 163 g
  Carbs: 213 g
  Fat: 44 g

  35% Protein
  45% Carbohydrates
  20% Fat

Marcella's Late Pre-Contest Meal Plan

Weight: 115 lbs
Body Fat: 14%

Meals and subsequent values varied day-to-day: calories, for example, varied between 1,100 and 1,350. These extremely low values were only maintained for the last few weeks before the contest. Refeed days of around 1,800 calories with extra carbohydrates and reduced fat and protein were eaten one day per week. Every other week this refeed day included a decadent meal out.

Breakfast:
¼ Block Extra Firm Tofu
¼ Bunch Broccoli, Cooked

Calories: 148
Protein: 14
Carbs: 13
Fat: 6

Post-Workout:
1 Scoop PlantFusion Protein

Calories: 120
Protein: 21
Carbs: 4
Fat: 2

Mid-Morning:
½ Scoop PlantFusion Protein
½ Cup Unsweetened Soymilk
1/8 Cup Cannellini Beans

Calories: 123
Protein: 16
Carbs: 8
Fat: 3

Lunch:

½ Head Romaine
Additional Raw Vegetable Salad Toppings (Cucumber, Tomato, Etc.)
¼ Block Extra Firm Tofu
Balsamic Vinegar

1 Bowl (About 1½ Cups) Red Lentil Soup
⅛ Bunch Broccoli, cooked

Calories: 324
Protein: 27
Carbs: 45
Fat: 7

Afternoon:
½ Scoop PlantFusion Protein
½ Cup Unsweetened Soymilk
1/8 Cup Cannellini Beans

Calories: 123
Protein: 16
Carbs: 8
Fat: 3

Dinner:
½ Head Romaine

¼ Block Extra Firm Tofu
3 Ounces Seitan
¼ Bunch Broccoli, Cooked

Calories: 369
Protein: 43
Carbs: 31
Fat: 11

Totals:

Calories: 1205
Protein: 138 g
Carbs: 109 g
Fat: 31 g

45% Protein
30% Carbohydrates
25% Fat

Appendix 2: Nutrition Guidelines, Menu Design, and Recipes

Our General Nutrition Guidelines

1. **Eat when you wake up**. This is very important because it stimulates your metabolism for the day and puts a stop to any muscle break down that may be occurring due to not having eaten in 8 or more hours.
2. **Eat every 2 to 3 hours**. This will keep our metabolic rate up all day (it takes energy to break down food) and will provide a steady stream of nutrients to keep energy levels up and food cravings at bay.
3. **Eat protein (beans, whole grains, nuts/seeds) and produce (fruits/veggies) at every meal/snack**. Protein is important for recovery and repair after exercise and keeps you feeling full, and produce is the healthiest food you can possibly eat since it's packed with vitamins, minerals, fiber, and antioxidants.
4. **Beans and greens are the top picks for protein and produce.** Both beans and leafy greens are packed with nutrients and are excellent sources of health-promoting energy. Eat them often - once a day at a minimum.
5. **Start lunch AND dinner with a big green salad.** Leafy greens and green vegetables are the most nutrient dense and health-promoting foods you can eat, so fill up on them first rather than less nutritious foods.
6. **Eat whole-food carbohydrates at most meals (whole grains, vegetables, fruit) and avoid refined carbohydrates (flour and sugar)**. Whole grains, fruits, and vegetables are extremely nutritious and their complex carbohydrates are exactly the type of fuel the human body is designed to thrive on for optimal health and peak performance. Refined carbohydrates are artificially condensed and rich, making them much more fattening, and are nearly devoid of nutrients after all the processing.

7. **Stop eating about 2 hours before bedtime**. When you sleep, your metabolic rate decreases, so going to bed with a belly full of calories may encourage some to be stored as body fat. Two hours is a good benchmark because that is the time it takes for most foods to move from the stomach to the small intestines, allowing you to go to bed with an 'empty' stomach.
8. **AVOID:**
   o Animal products, which contain the diet's only sources of cholesterol, saturated fat (almost), and animal protein. Each of these has been demonstrated to have very negative effects on long-term health.
   o Processed foods, (including ALL oils) which are stripped of nutrients, artificially calorie dense, and often contain toxic additives such as trans fats and high fructose corn syrup
   o Sodium, which in excess may cause damage to the vascular system and kidneys.

Menu Design

A guide to bodybuilding contest preparation wouldn't be complete without addressing the issue of meal planning! We've provided eight sample menus in this book, and more are available at our website and in articles we've written for veganbodybuilding.com. Any of these meal plans can be customized to your statistics, goals, and preferences with a little tweaking. Here are some suggestions:

- Non-starchy vegetables should never be limited! We don't bother tracking them or planning for them. For example, when Marcella makes a lentil soup that includes chopped celery and carrot, we don't bother tracking these vegetables in our food journals. It would be a lot of extra effort for something that makes very little difference in our calorie intake and macronutrient breakdown.

- Use a program that saves your previous entries rather than pencil and paper. We primarily use the Excel program Marcella created for this purpose, available for free download at our website as the "Free Diet Planner", because we can enter foods and recipes into it that we eat often and it is designed to show us exactly what we need: the macronutrient breakdown and calorie totals for each meal and for the day. It does require some familiarity with Excel. There are also a number of free online trackers and apps out there. CRON-O-Meter, for example, is very simple to use and is free to use at cronometer.com. You can search for videos detailing how to use it, but here is a basic overview:

  o You have to sign up. It will ask you to set a goal. Choose "Maintain weight". You can also set your preferred macronutrient ratio target, which you can choose to ignore but, if you like, you can enter a ratio. For example, entering "2:7:1" will set your preferred macronutrient ratio to 20% protein, 70% carbohydrates, and 10% fat.

  o Once in the Diary, you can click on the calories, protein, and other fields on the bottom and set targets. Choose a range for each that's around your targets.

  o You can then enter in all of the foods included in any of the above menus as your starting point, and begin playing around with them to create new menus by adding or deleting foods and changing quantities. As you change values, you can check the stats at the bottom of the page to make sure that you are still within your targets.

Meal planning gets easier with experience, especially as you can create a new menu from a previous menu that has worked for you in the past.

Recipes

As of this writing, Marcella has shared about 80 of her recipes on our website, so be sure to browse veganmuscleandfitness.com for additional ideas. We have also listed some of our favorite websites and cookbooks in Appendix 3. Here are a few of our staples.

Red Lentil Soup
Makes about 4 bowls.

Double the recipe for advance meal prep!

- o 1.5 cups dried red lentils
- o 2 cloves crushed or minced garlic
- o 4.5 cups water
- o 2 tsp curry powder (optional)
- o 1/8 cup ume vinegar, found in Asian or International aisle (optional)
- o 1 Tbsp ginger paste or minced ginger (optional)
- o 2 cups chopped broccoli and carrots (optional)

In a pot, bring lentils, garlic, and water to a boil. Turn down to medium-low, cover, and simmer for 20 minutes.

Stir in curry powder, vinegar, and ginger and simmer 5 minutes.

Serve with a baked sweet potato and a large green salad topped with blackened tofu for our standard contest prep lunch!

Blackened Tofu

Makes enough to top four salads.

- o   1 block extra firm tofu
- o   1 to 2 tsp preferred seasoning, such as Blackened Creole, Cajun, or Jamaican jerk
- o   nutritional yeast
- o   salt or cooking spray

Dice or slice the tofu into strips. Preheat a pan on medium high and sprinkle with a bit of salt or spray briefly with cooking spray to keep the tofu from sticking.

Toss the tofu on, and let it "blacken" a bit on one side. Add seasoning, then flip over and toss around, preferably with a metal spatula to get under the tofu without any sticking to the pan. Sprinkle with nutritional yeast, flip and cook a little more, then serve over salad.

Southern Beans and Greens Bowl

Makes two generous dinners. Serve in salad bowls!

- o   2 cups of uncooked rice, cooked
- o   ½ onion diced
- o   1 stalk celery. minced
- o   2 tsp Cajun or Blackened Creole seasoning
- o   1 can diced tomatoes, drained
- o   1 cube vegan bouillon, no salt added (Rapunzel is a good brand)
- o   Chopped collards, kale, or mustard greens with stems removed

- o   1 ½ cup cooked or 1 can black-eyed peas
     or pinto beans
- o   ½ avocado, chopped (optional)

In a large saucepan, sauté onions and celery in a bit of water on medium-high heat for 5 minutes. Add seasoning, tomatoes, bouillon cube, and ¼ cup water. Stir.

Add greens, cover, and simmer on medium-low for about 10 minutes.

Add beans, stir, cover, and simmer again for about 10 minutes.

Serve over rice and top with avocado.

Appendix 3: Resources

Recipe Sources

www.veganmuscleandfitness.com
www.happyherbivore.com/recipes
www.straightupfood.com
www.forksoverknives.com/recipes
www.theppk.com
www.eatunprocessed.com/dietitian.html

Fitness and Nutrition Resources

www.veganmuscleandfitness.com
www.veganbodybuilding.com
www.facebook.com/groups/VeganBodybuildingAndFitness/
www.youtube.com/user/Veganmusclenfitness
http://www.exrx.net/

Documentaries

Forks Over Knives
Planeat
Vegucated
Cowspiracy: The Sustainability Secret
Earthlings
Speciesim: The Movie

Recommended Reading

Vegan Bodybuilding & Fitness: The Complete Guide to Building Your Body on a Plant-Based Diet by Robert Cheeke

Shred It! The Vegan Bodybuilding & Fitness Guide to Burning Fat and Building Muscle by Robert Cheeke

The Complete Idiot's Guide to Plant-Based Nutrition by Julieanna Hever M.S., R.D., C.P.T.

Disease-Proof Your Child: Feeding Kids Right by Dr. Joel Fuhrman

Forks Over Knives: The Plant-Based Way to Health by Dr. T. Colin Campbell and Dr. Caldwell B. Esselstyn, Jr.

Unprocessed: How to achieve vibrant health and your ideal weight by Chef AJ and Glen Merzer

Breaking the Food Seduction: The Hidden Reasons Behind Food Cravings and 7 Steps to End Them Naturally by Dr. Neal D. Barnard

Foods That Cause You to Lose Weight: The Negative Calorie Effect by Dr. Neal Barnard

The Engine 2 Diet: The Texas Firefighter's 28-Day Save-Your-Life Plan that Lowers Cholesterol and Burns Away the Pounds by Rip Esselstyn

21-Day Weight Loss Kickstart: Boost Metabolism, Lower Cholesterol, and Dramatically Improve Your Health by Dr. Neal Barnard

Keep It Simple, Keep It Whole: Your Guide To Optimum Health by Dr. Alona Pulde and Dr. Matthew Lederman

The Get Healthy, Go Vegan Cookbook: 125 Easy and Delicious Recipes to Jump-Start Weight Loss and Help You Feel Great by Dr. Neal Barnard

Prevent and Reverse Heart Disease: The Revolutionary, Scientifically Proven, Nutrition-Based Cure by Dr. Caldwell B. Esselstyn Jr.

Dr. Neal Barnard's Program for Reversing Diabetes: The Scientifically Proven System for Reversing Diabetes without Drugs by Dr. Neal D. Barnard

Appetite for Reduction: 125 Fast and Filling Low-Fat Vegan Recipes by Isa Chandra Moskowitz

Forks Over Knives - The Cookbook: Over 300 Recipes for Plant-Based Eating All Through the Year by Del Sroufe

And any other titles by the above authors!

Thank You for Reading!

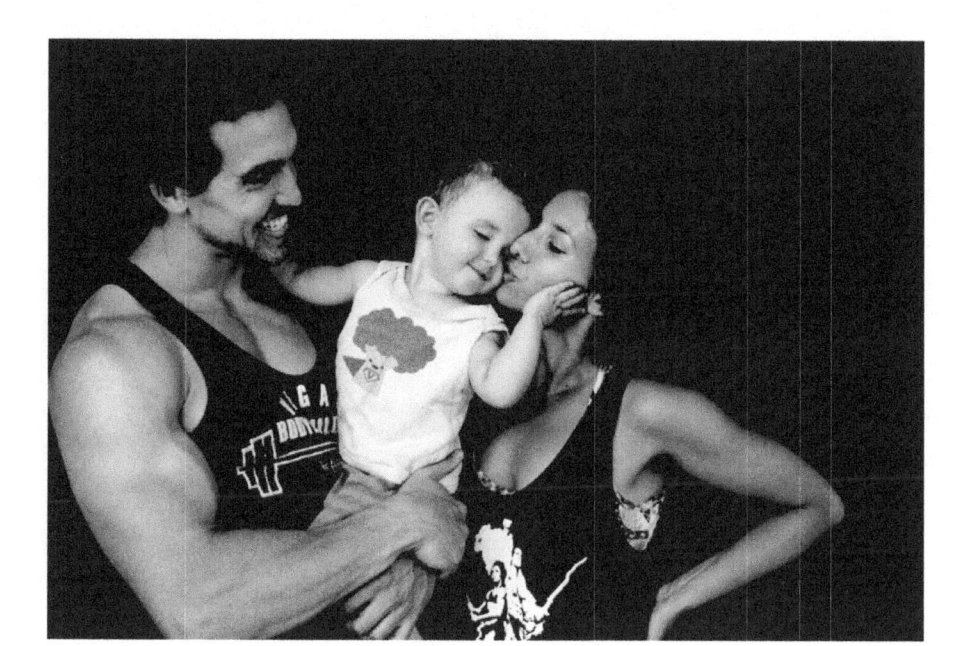

Photo by Melissa Schwartz

Made in the USA
Las Vegas, NV
07 October 2021

31888325R00080